Well, I'

Joanne Gillespie is a pupil at Grangefield School in Stockton-on-Tees. Despite the fact that her really cruel father has a car she has to walk there every day carrying lots of books, PE kit and a packed lunch. She gets far too much homework, which she feels is a serious distraction from *Home and Away* and *Neighbours*. She will be sixteen on 5 December 1993 (seventeen on 5 December 1994 – just in case family or friends forget!).

She intends to own a bright red sports car one day, enjoys books, loud music, ballet and the theatre – AND FRESH CREAM CAKES! She hates carrot juice, alarm clocks, walking to school and cigarette smoke.

She lives with her parents and sister, all of whom she loves very much. She loves life itself, red skies, rain clouds, full moons and knows how lucky she has been.

Well, I'm Still Here!

JOANNE GILLESPIE

Celebrating five years clear of cancer

ILLUSTRATED BY
SARAH GILLESPIE

Pan

First published 1993 by
Pan Macmillan Children's Books
a division of Pan Macmillan Publishers Limited
Cavaye Place London SW10 9PG
and Basingstoke

Associated companies throughout the world

ISBN 0 330 32714 3

Illustrations by Sarah Gillespie

1 3 5 7 9 8 6 4 2

A CIP catalogue record for this book is available from
the British Library

Typeset by Cambridge Composing (UK) Limited, Cambridge
Printed in England by Cox and Wyman Limited

TO IZZY,

THANK YOU FOR BEING A FRIEND

Introduction

Imagine you are writing a poem entitled 'I Wish'. You can wish for anything you want. How would you start it? How would you finish it? Win the pools? Play for England? Marry a prince?

Now imagine you've been seriously ill, you've had two brain tumours, radiotherapy has left you bald, you've almost doubled your weight because of steroid tablets, you've had a stroke and your arm and leg are paralysed. Now, write that same poem and what do you wish for?

This was the state of my daughter's health when she was ten years old and decided to write a poem called 'I Wish'.

How would you start it?

Her poem began . . .

> *'I wish that all the wars would end,*
> *That every person could be a friend'*

and ended . . .

> *'I wish everyone was as happy as I am'*

Not once did she complain about her health or wish it had happened to someone else.

Nor did she wish that it had never happened. Obviously, she wanted to be better, but that was going to take courage and determination. She believed in God, but that's not always enough; God wants us to believe in ourselves, then when we are working together anything can happen! These are Joanne's words, not mine, but just because they come from a child doesn't mean they are not true.

Joanne was born in 1977, an only child until 1981, when her sister Sarah Jane was born. Her life revolved around dancing and telling jokes. That sense of humour and love of dance were to be of great help to her and to us in the years that lay ahead.

In 1986 Joanne was diagnosed as having a brain tumour. For a few weeks before that fateful Friday, when we were given the news, she had been suffering severe headaches, sickness and dizziness, which our doctor put down to migraine. He prescribed medication and warned us of its side effects. Joanne suddenly suffered paralysis down the right-hand side of her body. Peter, her father, wondered if he had given her the wrong amount of medication and if that had caused the problem. We went to our doctor, who decided to send Joanne for further tests at our local hospital. By the time we arrived at the hospital, she was starting to feel better and was once again telling jokes. We were now worried that if they sent her home too early, they would still not find out exactly what was wrong with her.

Only a parent who is told that their child has a life-threatening disease can truly know how we felt. The words CANCER, BRAIN TUMOUR or MENINGITIS were thought to be the probable causes of her illness. Can you imagine sitting in a doctor's office, wondering which one of these three diseases you would rather your child has? You keep thinking it is all a big mistake and it won't be any of these three, that you can go home and everything will be all right.

Words became a jumble, we were numb, it was as if we were in a different place and that it was happening to someone else. We didn't take in everything he said, only odd words filtered through. We seemed to be in a dream. We wanted to get out of the office as quickly as possible. How dare he talk about our child like that! What had we ever done to deserve this? It was unfair – *life* was unfair – God was unfair. Why not someone else's child? Anybody's but our lovely little girl. We hope God forgives us now for thinking like that, but you suddenly become irrational and all sense goes. Far from being unfair, God has helped us get through the last six years, for without His help and strength we would never have been able to cope.

Acting as though nothing was wrong, but with a dead feeling inside, we told Joanne she would have to move hospitals so she could have a brain scan, which would tell the doctors exactly what was going on in her head. The reason for the move was that our local hospital did not have the equipment and the nearest was Middlesbrough General. It was here we met Mr Nath for the first time. He was to become both our's and Joanne's friend, as well as her brain surgeon. It may seem strange to become friendly with the man who may one day have to tell you that he can do no more for your child, but his honesty, even at the cruellest moments, was appreciated.

The diagnosis was confirmed after the scan and the operation was scheduled for the following Tuesday. There was only a 60/40 per cent chance of her coming through the operation as she was so weak. The operation lasted five hours, and they were the longest five hours of our lives. She came through, she seemed fine and was allowed home only six days later, on our thirteenth wedding anniversary. Mr Nath told us it was thought to be a benign tumour and because of her weak state he could not remove it all. However, it was probably a slow-growing tumour and would not recur until she was a teenager. By that time more advances in medicine would have been made, so we thought everything would be fine.

During the next few months Joanne returned to school and to dancing: everything was going to be all right.

Joanne and Sarah were given the opportunity to perform in our local Stage Society's production of *The King and I* in about February 1987. We found out later that Joanne had started suffering headaches again. She didn't tell us in case we decided to take her out of the show. She performed really well and enjoyed every minute. She covered up the pain she was feeling, until it became obvious something was seriously wrong: the headaches came closer together and the sickness started again. We took her back to the doctor, but deep down we knew the worst was happening. We contacted Mr Nath direct and he told us to bring her straight in and he would do another brain scan. Mr Nath was in the operating theatre for the rest of the day and was unable to look at the scan to tell us the result. We waited at the hospital until 9 p.m., when the house doctor said that Mr Nath had been delayed and told us to go home. He said, 'Don't quote me, but I've looked at the scan and I think it's clear.' We felt uplifted, and went home happy. After spending the evening phoning family to tell them the good news, we opened a bottle of wine to celebrate. The moment we put the phone down, it rang. It was Mr Nath to say he'd been trying to phone all evening to tell us the tumour was back.

It was the worst time of all. To be told everything was OK, to have our spirits lifted and then for our hopes to be dashed was absolutely terrible. Peter went to pieces. I didn't know what to do, our world seemed to be ending all over again. I telephoned our minister and he was round within minutes and stayed with us for hours, helping us through the worst.

We went back to hospital the next morning and saw Mr Nath who told us the position and that he would have to operate again. This time he thought her chances of paralysis were greatly increased, but felt he had to give her every chance.

We had already arranged two family trips. One to Scarborough that weekend to see *Swan Lake*, and a holiday to Menorca the following week. Mr Nath told us to go ahead with both, as they would probably be the last family trips which Joanne, if she survived the operation, would be able to really enjoy, as she could suffer paralysis or loss of speech.

The trip to Scarborough went ahead the following day. Joanne sat watching her beloved ballet, while we sat watching the dying swan and took advantage of the time to cry.

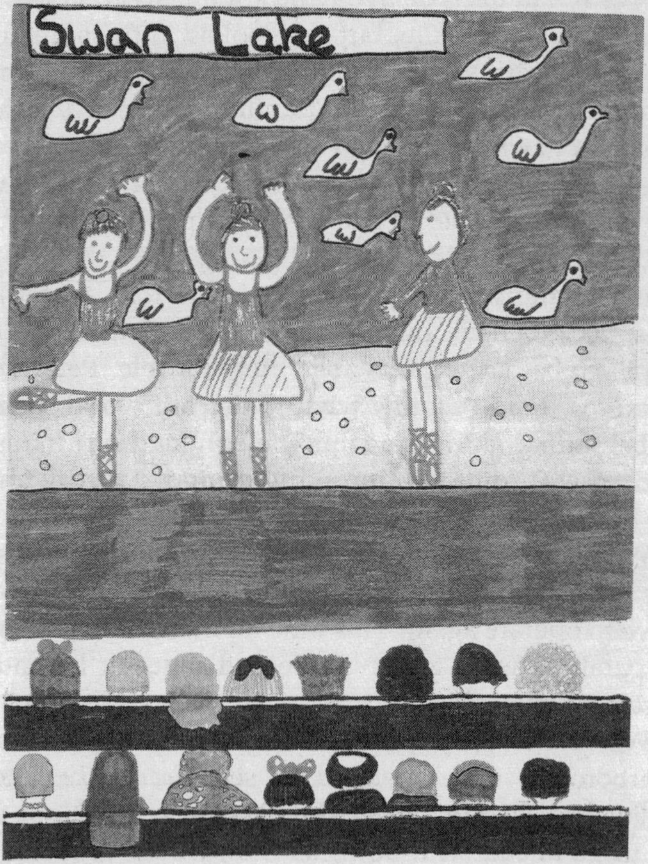

In Menorca, Joanne danced every night. We sat watching her, thinking of what lay ahead for us when we returned home and wondering if we would ever see her dance again. On the last night she was presented with a medal by the holiday representative for her excellent dancing all that week. This was lovely for Joanne but only added to our heartache.

The operation was arranged for Tuesday and we were told it would last approximately the same length of time as the first, which was five hours. In fact it took over seven hours! She came out of the operating theatre and was returned to Intensive Care where she was wrapped in silver foil to keep in her body heat. The doctors wanted to know if her memory, speech or any part of her body had been affected by their tampering with her brain for over seven hours. They asked what her name was and she said, 'Joanne Louise Gillespie.' We smiled – she never uses her middle name. 'Do you know where you are?' they asked, expecting her to say 'in hospital'. She said, 'I'm in Intensive Care, in Ward 9.' We smiled again. They began to prod her, asking if she could feel anything. First her left hand, arm, then foot – everytime asking if she could feel anything. We smiled when she said yes to her hand, again when she said yes to her arm, and when asked about her foot, she said, 'Of course I can, they didn't operate on my feet, they did it on my head, stupid!' We actually laughed out loud. They then started on the right-hand side of her body. Wherever they touched there was no feeling. We stopped smiling.

FEAR

Fear is the day before the operation

Wondering what might happen

Fear is the day of the operation

Getting wheeled down to the theatre

I was clinging on my mam's hand but I had to leave my parents behind

I saw the doctors & nurses with masks on

FEAR IS THE UNKNOWN

The tumour had spread considerably, much more than was first thought. Mr Nath told us afterwards that it had spread so far and was so malignant that he did not hold out much hope, and thought that within six months it would grow again and there was very little he could do. A course of radiotherapy was planned. A mask had to be made of Joanne's head. This meant covering her face in plaster. Her eyes, ears and mouth were covered – only her nose was left, so that she could breathe. She had to lie perfectly still until the plaster dried. She held very tightly on to Peter and I. Despite being afraid she knew it was very important that the mask fitted perfectly to get the maximum benefit. We were told afterwards that many adults panic when their senses are cut off and several attempts are needed to make a mask that fits correctly. Joanne only needed one. She was given the mask after the treatment finished, and she uses it to keep her hat and sunglasses on.

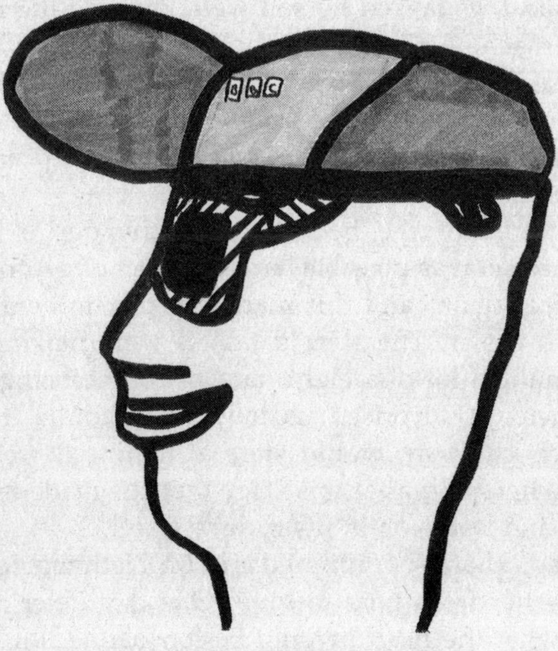

How Long Is Two Weeks?

How long is two weeks?
Why is my hair falling out
What are steroids for
Why am I fat
Will my sister be alright
Are you still there mum
When can we go home
HOW LONG IS TWO WEEKS

The treatment made all of Joanne's hair fall out, apart from a little bit at the front and back. She did not suffer from sickness during that time, as she stayed very positive and visualized herself well, imaging the radiotherapy machine wiping out the bad cells in her body. Her sense of humour helped her too – telling the nurses jokes and helping to serve tea and biscuits to the other patients. She was determined not to give up and to prove the doctors wrong.

Her hatred of the bed pan and the desire to be dancing as soon as possible had the effect of getting her on her feet again, and this made the physiotherapist's job much easier. The steroid tablets were making her put on quite a lot of weight, and of course being bald didn't help. It surprised us that many adults, rather than their children, would stare at Joanne if we took her anywhere. It was at this stage that she made herself a badge and wrote on it 'It's rude to stare!'

The radiotherapy continued and Mr Nath would pop in to see her from time to time. One day Peter asked exactly what the future would be for Joanne. Mr Nath replied 'Not good.' 'But the operation, the radiotherapy?' Peter said. Mr Nath answered that some surgeons would not have carried out the operation a second time, since the tumour had returned within one year, but he had felt that Joanne deserved the chance of everything that was medically available. Being realistic, he thought she might live until Christmas, but not Easter. 'Not any chance at all?' Peter asked. 'What do you want me to say?' he said. 'One in a million, probably more.' Peter kept telling himself Mr Nath was wrong, and anyway,

THE SCARECROW

I am a scarecrow and that is all

I frighten birdies big and small

The crows are crafty......but just one look at me

And they fly with fear back to the family

I enjoy my job very much

But every day I'm thinking of a way to look handsome and pretty, in a

scarecrow sort of way

But at the moment I look awful with my twig fingers and curly carrot nose

And especially my root-sprouting chin

Oh, well, I give in

I'll keep the sprouting root chin

I don't care what I look like - because.......

What counts is what your like WITHIN!!!

one in a million was better than no chance at all. 'Look,' Mr Nath spoke again, 'to have any chance at all, Joanne has to have five years completely clear of cancer, but you have to understand that's not going to happen.'

When Joanne was asleep, Peter told me what Mr Nath had said. We sat in Joanne's bedroom and decided who we would invite to the big party we were going to have in 1992, to celebrate Joanne's five years clear of cancer!

It seemed that every time someone said something negative it made us more determined to be positive. Joanne was following the Bristol Diet, taking multi-vitamins and had joined a self-help group. We were investigating different therapies and our family were writing letters to people all over the world trying to find out what medical expertise was available, and where. Then one day, shortly after the radiotherapy finished, Joanne was sitting watching TV when she began behaving very oddly. She started making uncontrollable movements and was unable to speak. She grabbed at the table for a pen, but the movements got stronger, and we soon realized that they had a pattern to them. For a second we thought she was mucking about. Half a second later I was phoning the hospital and Peter was fastening Joanne's seat belt – and belting down the road to the hospital. Once again, the doctors and nurses were incredible; so, I must add, was Sarah, who although very young at the time helped her sister during what seemed to be a fit. Joanne screamed with pain all night and everyone did all they could to help.

The next day the results of her tests showed that she had had a stroke, not a fit. We were told a blood vessel in her head had collapsed, probably as a result of the radiotherapy. The right-hand side of Joanne's body was paralysed again. For a third time her determination to dance would be tested. She told us afterwards that that was the most scared she had ever been. She had wanted to speak but had been unable to and had made a grab for the pen to write 'HELP', but couldn't control her arms. Despite regular physiotherapy, Joanne has never fully recovered the use of her right arm and hand; she still suffers from painful spasms all the way down to her fingers. The strength came back into her leg, although she walked with difficulty for quite some time.

Joanne was absent from school and feeling bored. She had tried to read the books that we had about cancer, but couldn't understand them. She decided to write a book for other children who were suffering from cancer, so that they wouldn't be afraid and would understand what was going on.

We wanted her to exercise her arm as much as possible, and encouraged her to colour in some of the drawings she had made in hospital. When she decided it was finished, we sent it to lots of different publishers but no one was interested in it. Then Suzanne Kruger, who ran the then Children's Cancer Help Centre, asked if she could use some of it in the monthly newsletter, and shortly afterwards a researcher from the BBC contacted us and asked if Joanne would appear on *Wogan*, when she felt well enough.

Joanne did appear on the programme and the interview went really well. Terry asked her to read a passage from her book. She read, 'Crying. Crying is all right and you have got to do it sometimes, but please don't cry all the time . . .' Terry said she was very brave, fighting back against cancer. Joanne replied, 'Cancer will never kill me. If I die, it will be because God wants me.'

Joanne's first book, *Brave Heart*, was published in 1989 and this, her second book, tells of her determination to achieve five years clear of cancer, against all the odds!

KATHY GILLESPIE

Joanne's Introduction

Hi, I'm Joanne. Not many laughs in the first chapter. That was my mam and dad's experience. Well, this is my story, so I'm taking over now. This is how it goes:

I was sick, I got better and
intend to stay that way!
THE END.

Not quite enough? Well . . . OK, I'll fill you in on all the details, but before I do I had better give you the low-down on my family. I live in a total madhouse, with three weirdos.

My mam (Kathy), my dad (Peter) and my sister (Sarah – or 'Spam', 'Sags' or 'Spamaloso', whichever my dad decides to call her at the time). My dad's like that. When my hair was just starting to grow back again after the radiotherapy, he called me 'Spike'. When we realized my poorly hand wasn't growing the same as my left hand, he called me 'Clock' (because I had one hand bigger than the other!). In between he called me 'Spud', but mostly he says, 'Hi, love.'

So we start with Dad . . . My dad is a strange mixture, sometimes he is like a strict headmaster, but mostly he is a complete nutter! He wanders around the house singing or shouting, 'YO DUDE! GIVE ME SOME SKIN!' and then he pretends we slap his hands too hard. He is convinced he is a Patrick Swayze/Tom Cruise look-alike and has now started imitating Arnold Schwarzenegger. He always starts when *Neighbours* or anything else he considers boring is on TV with shouts of 'Asta Lavista, Baby!' He tickles or pesters Mam, Sarah or me until we are all screaming at him to leave us alone, but, just like big Arnie, we know HE WILL BE BACK! IRRITATOR 2, the Judgement Day, that's Dad.

Of course, like most dads it's different when there's sport on TV, especially football, cricket or golf. He really likes golf, although he is hopeless at it and loses loads of balls. One year for Christmas, Sarah and I bought him some golf-ball soaps, which we put into the soap box in the bathroom. Eventually the day came when a new bar of soap was needed. Dad, who is blind as a bat without his glasses, fumbled around in the box for soap and eventually grabbed our present. He later pretended to stop our pocket money . . . You see, we put real golf balls in the box and Dad had been scrubbing his body with them, trying to get a lather!

One thing that *does* get Dad into a lather is anyone who he thinks is being unfair or unpleasant to Sarah or me. At times like this, it's best to keep out of his way. When his temper goes, it really goes . . . The funny thing is, no matter how bad-tempered he gets, it only takes him a minute and he is his old silly self again.

So! That's my dad! Average height, getting a bit of a tummy, short-sighted and always wears bright coloured clothes . . . Sounds just like Patrick Swayze, doesn't he?

But he still gives me a kiss each night at bedtime, pretends he's tough and that things don't bother him (though I know that's not true), and, despite all his faults, I want to marry someone just like him.

So, what about Mam? Well, Mam's brill too! She is much quieter than Dad, but so are most people. Our main link with sanity, Mam always seems to understand. When I was in hospital we told each other secrets and now I find it easy to talk to her about anything, especially girls' stuff. Like most mums she has some crazy ideas, like *keep your room tidy* and *don't leave dirty clothes on the floor, put them in the linen bin*! Sarah and me call her the 'Tidy Police' and Dad calls her 'the old bird'. She can be moody, and although she doesn't get as bad-tempered as Dad, her moods seem to last longer! She likes all the soaps on TV and Tom Jones, and her ambition is to ride in a helicopter. She works as a typist for Stockton Council and spends every weekend catching up on housework. She hates ironing, but does it anyway; she can drive but never does. She is determined to learn to swim, though it may take quite a long time! I suppose she is like lots of other people's mums, but she is special . . . She is MY MAM.

The other weirdo in our house is my sister Sarah. Sarah is eleven. Sometimes she pretends to be really shy. She has the face of an angel and the mind of a skinhead – a complete thug. She always has a secret stash of chocolate upstairs, despite what Mam says. She draws really good pictures, is brilliant on the organ and keyboard and fights with me over everything, especially whose turn it is to choose a video on our family afternoons each Sunday, when we all settle down to watch TV. Sometimes I think, 'Right, pal, you're for it this time,' and it's incredible, every time I am just about to thump her, Dad walks in and catches me! Whenever she bugs me and I tell Dad, she looks ever so innocent and Dad says, 'Don't fight, girls.' But I'll tell you this, however much I fight with my sister, we always look out for each other and I am sure if you have a smaller brother or sister, they can be a real pain in the neck, but I think Sarah is just the way I would have been at ten if I had never had cancer.

People

TERRY WOGAN's really very nice,
I've been on his chat show, in fact I've been on twice
I stayed with JEFF BANKS from 'The Clothes Show'
Played with Coco and India and met his wife SUE
Their house is really gorgeous
And has a big posh loo
SHAKIN' STEVENS, BONNIE LANGFORD,
She let me wear her hat,
'Me and My Girl' was brilliant
and we had a lovely chat
I've met a real live Royal Duchess

and danced with The Northern Ballet
I've spoken for God at The Albert Hall
and at Westminster Abbey
I've met some really lovely folk
But I'll tell you who's the best
A person who can be a pain, a proper little pest
I see her every morning and she gives my arm a tug
She's my sister Sarah, she's 8 and she's a thug
But times when I've been poorly
and some friends ran away,
My sister, she stayed with me
SHE'S A STAR – THAT'S WHAT I SAY!!

Of course, leaving the best till last, there is also me. I am tall, slim, fantastically good-looking, modest and always telling lies! Well, to be honest, I am a little bit overweight, and try as I do, eating all the right things, one of the side effects of my tablets is weight gain. I'm on the smaller side of average height – *that's* my problem you see, I'm not really overweight just under-tall! I like really bright clothes and although much of my hair has grown back, I still have a large bald patch – I call it my 'sun roof' – on the top of my head. I love dancing, Michael Jackson and the occasional cream cake. I am told I'm a mother hen, I like looking after babies, I worry about the environment, I think smoking is disgusting and I have taught myself to write left-handed (my right hand isn't very good). I enjoy drama and am becoming aware that the early sympathy felt for me is changing to jealousy and dislike. I know who my really good friends are. I can be bossy but that comes from my determination to get what I want. I get far too much homework and not nearly enough pocket money and I still get tired very easily. With the exception of a few boys in the fourth and fifth year, I think most of the boys in my school are wimps, but the best ones never seem to fancy me! I think I am OK, just like everyone else, but I am not in so many different ways.

Friends

Friends are people who will always be near
They won't run away in times of fear
But some friends are fickle, they soon disappear
Don't get upset – they aren't worth the tear.

So that's my family – four people who do everything together, laugh, cry, play or fight. No favourites, no special treatment, just us. Some days I can't get home from school quick enough. I know I'll have homework to do, but I feel much happier at home. Some people say I had to grow up very quickly, but I know there's a lot of love in my house, and I don't think it's childish to still want a cuddle from Mam or Dad.

Although Mam and Dad had always promised me that they would tell me no lies, they didn't promise me they would tell me the whole truth, and so they never told me that the doctors thought I only had six months to live, because I never asked. I had had my two operations, finished the course of radiotherapy and had had a stroke, and at that point, knowing that there was little more the doctors could do for me, Mam and Dad decided to find out about alternative therapies. They travelled all over the country and read all sorts of books, and eventually we settled on the Bristol Cancer Diet Programme. This meant I had to take lots of different vitamins and drink lots of carrot juice, etc. That wasn't very nice, so, as an encouragement, they said that if I stayed with it for a year, then instead of having to go back to hospital in April (as I had done for the two previous years), they would take me to America, to Disneyland! This seemed a much better idea than being in hospital and so, obviously, I agreed. The condition was that I had to stay well; if I did happen to become ill again, the doctors wouldn't let me travel. I didn't know at this point that Mam and Dad were planning this for six months after the time the doctors gave me, that's the kind of sneaky people they are. They planned little things for me – some things quite close, some things in the future. Something for me to look forward to all the time. So, as the picnics, trips to the ballet, etc, passed by, and America got gradually nearer, we eventually reached Christmas.

Christmas is always a special time in our house, it's brilliant. I suppose it must have been especially brilliant and especially sad, in a funny kind of way, for Mam and Dad, knowing now that this would probably be the last Christmas I would ever have with them. Again, they didn't let me know that. Christmas that year was absolutely *magic*.

Another couple of months went by and it was February. It was winter. As a one-time bald person, I can tell you it's not funny being without hair in the winter! It's really cold. I had a range of hats and scarves. I didn't like wigs, people laughed at me when I wore them and laughed at me when I kept them off. My hair was starting to grow through a little bit and Dad now started calling me 'Baldylocks'. He always comes up with something or other. The snow disappeared and gradually leaves and blossom appeared back on the trees in our garden. It was almost time to go to Disneyland. I had to go to see Mr Nath again to get a special letter to say that I was able to travel, and in case anything happened to me while I was abroad. Nothing did, but we had to be covered anyway.

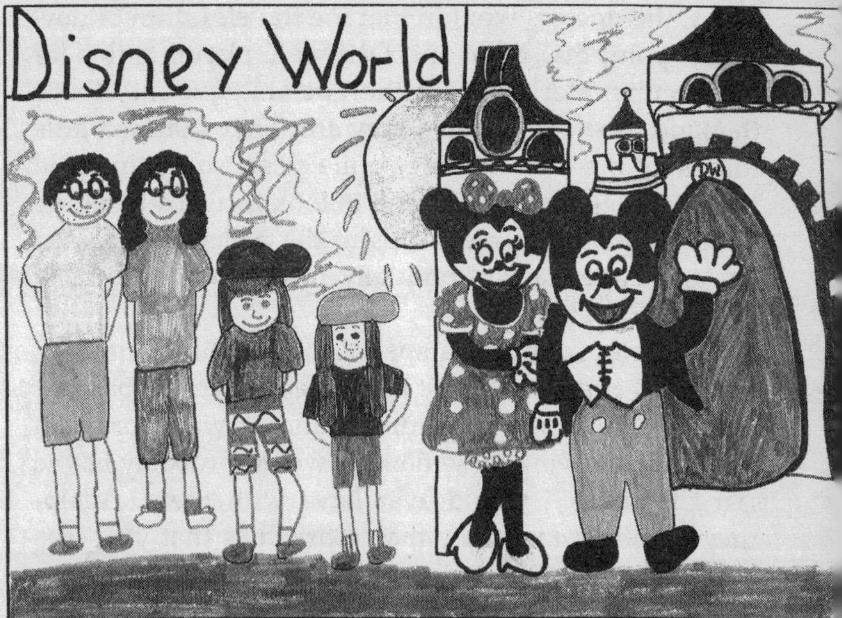

We went to America and it was fabulous. The sunshine, hotel, swimming pool, Disneyland, Mickey Mouse, Epcot Centre . . . everything was brill. When we got back home, Dad said to me, 'The doctors said you would never live long enough to go on that journey.' I didn't understand what he meant – I looked at Mam and she said, 'That's right.' Dad said to me that they were told I would be paralysed, *but you're not*; they were told I might never speak again, *but you can*; and they were told that I would never be able to dance, *but you do*, so what are you going to do now? They have said you're going to die – are you going to do it, and prove them right? Or do you want to stay around a little longer, do a few more things, go back to Disneyland, be really awkward and prove them wrong? We all sat together and cried. After a while I thought . . . NO, I'M NOT GOING TO DIE. I WANT TO LIVE. NO WAY, I'M NOT GOING TO DIE. I WANT TO LIVE, I'M GOING TO LIVE! – I'LL SHOW THEM.

BEST DECISION I EVER MADE . . .

Hi, im Sarah, i'm 10 now and i'm Joannes Sister. I was only 5 when Joanne was first taken into hospital. I didn't know What Cancer was, but I Could See that it made grown-ups Scared. Joanne didn't have Spots or anything, and She seemed alright, so I was quite angry That she got lots of attention and presents of people and I had to go to School everyday. The Worst thing was that my mam Spent every day and night with Joanne in hospital, and although dad Came home on a night and I could in his bedroom with him, I Spent most of my time with my nana.

My nana's nice, but I wanted my mam and dad back. I suppose I started thinking that they loved her more than me. When Joanne came home mam and dad tried really hard to make me feel special, But it wasn't the same because Joanne was there and I wanted them just for me, like Joanne had. It wasn't until I saw Joanne having a fit that I knew that she wasn't kidding and something was really wrong with her. When she came out of hospital again, she could hardly use her arm or leg.

Sometimes Joanne is a pain

in the neck. She can be very bossy and not very good to play with. Sometimes she used to moan that I wouldn't give her a kiss or if she offered a bite of ice cream or something, I would say no. Because I saw adults afraid of cancer, I thought I could catch it off her. Now I know that I can't, and noone can, we play much better. I Love my Sister and she loves me, I know that though Sometimes I don't show it, and I don't ever want her to be poorly again.

THE OCTOPUS

Squidgy and Squirmy
Green, Huge and Ugly
Its slippery smooth skin
Then his eight arms begin
His evil looking eyes glare at me
Oh my gosh! Does he want me for his tea?
He sneakily hides from his prey - That is the
day of the Octopus
He squirts black ink in my face, his strong arms
squeeze round me,
I try to fight this Octopus but he's a deadly
enemy.
Grasping and wriggling I worked my way free
I get in my little boat -
This Octopus is Never again going to see me!

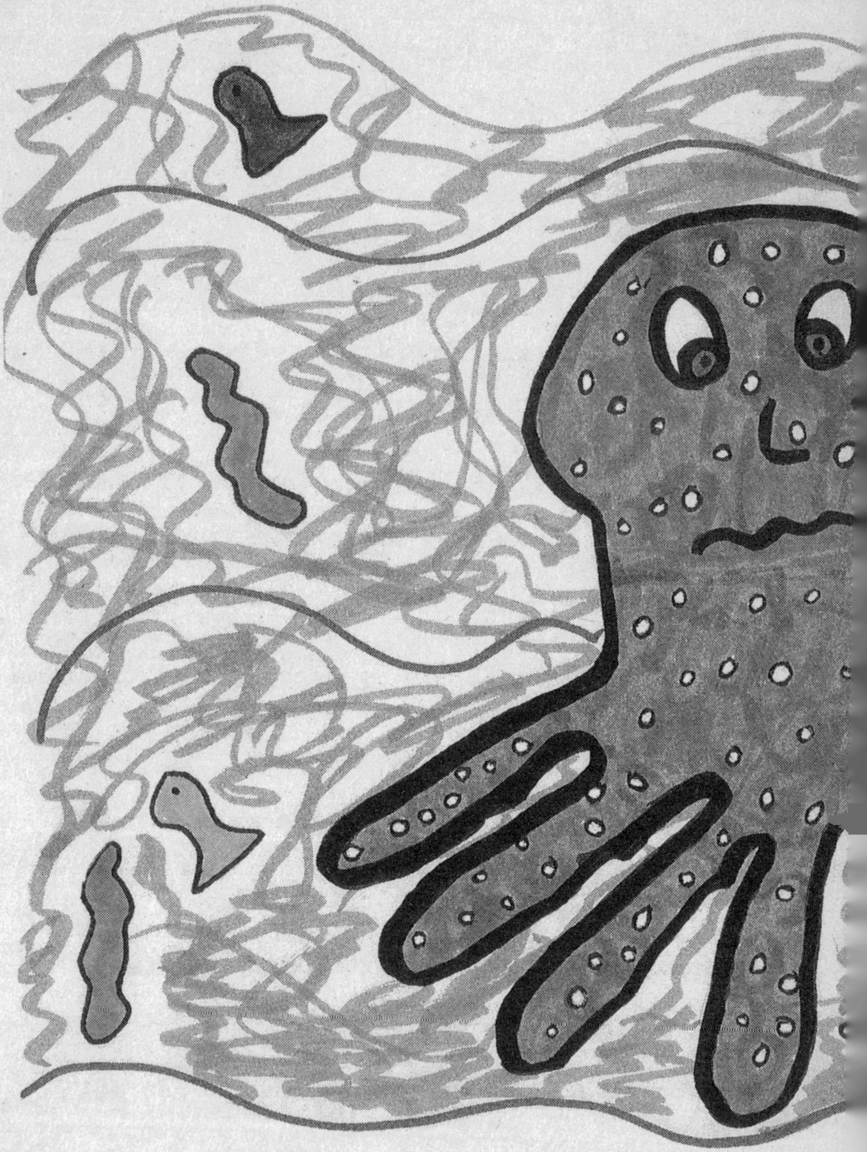

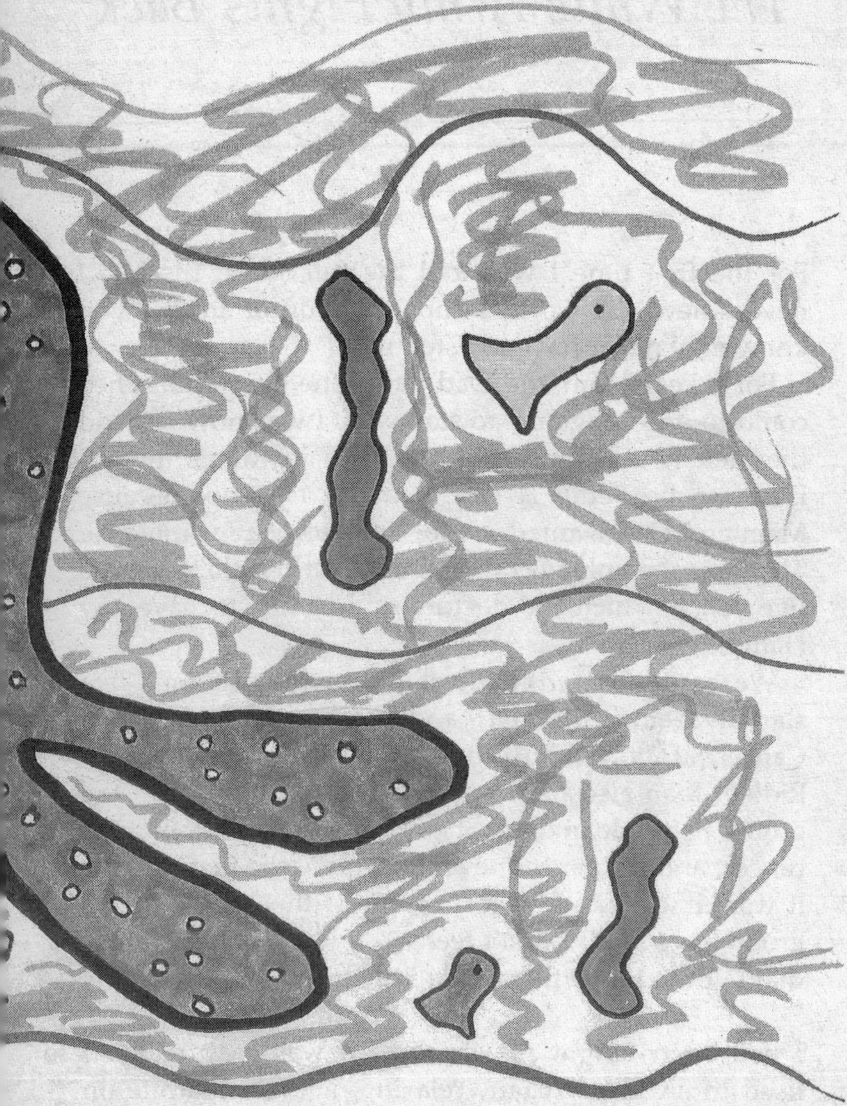

The White Army Fights Back

For the first time I was told the full story, the bits I never knew, the words I hope that you or anyone you know may never have to listen to.

For a year Mam and Dad had done everything they could to encourage me to stay well. I was now ten and they felt it was time I took a hand in things myself. I had to be better *because I wanted to* – not because Mam and Dad wanted me to, but because *I* wanted to. That was the only way they knew that I could reach the five years, which the doctors said I must to have any chance.

We continued with the diet and the vitamins, we started seeing a healer, and we started going to a Cancer Support Group run by a lovely lady called Joan Ridley. Joan also had cancer, like all the others in the group. Sadly, Joan died. She never stopped fighting the cancer, and the cancer never beat her – she just decided it was time to have a rest. A lot of the people in the group have died. I don't feel sad, I just feel I was lucky that I got to know them for a little time.

I had been taught to visualize; it was easy really. I used to sit in my chair, relaxing, and concentrate on something that I really wanted to happen. I had been told that everyone has in their blood white cells. It's these white cells that help us to get better when we have a cut or anything. I decided to visualize white cells in my body, not just one or two – *millions* of super-fit white cells: THE WHITE ARMY! I would concentrate on this white army going to my brain and surrounding and completely killing anything that was grey. The grey areas I saw as the tumour – the white army would smash, rip, tear and completely kill all of the tumour away from my body. I would finish by thinking of a waterfall. The water would run right through my body and clear away all the dead cells, leaving only the white cells to protect me against cancer ever coming back.

By the time I was invited on to *Wogan* I was feeling a lot better. My hair was growing quite nicely now. I had recovered quite a lot of use in my leg, my arm was still pretty useless but I felt quite good. We set off from Darlington station for London. It was a bit embarrassing really, nearly all the local newspapers had a picture of me, saying that I was going to be on *Wogan*. I could see the people in the train looking at the newspapers and glancing up at me, looking at the paper again. I felt like shouting, 'YES, FOLKS – IT'S ME!' Modesty has never been one of my strong points!

When we got off the train there was a chauffeur waiting to take us to our hotel. It was really posh. When we got to the hotel there were loads of journalists waiting to see me as we went in; I felt just like Madonna! We were taken to the BBC and I was escorted to my dressing room – DRESSING ROOM NO. 3.

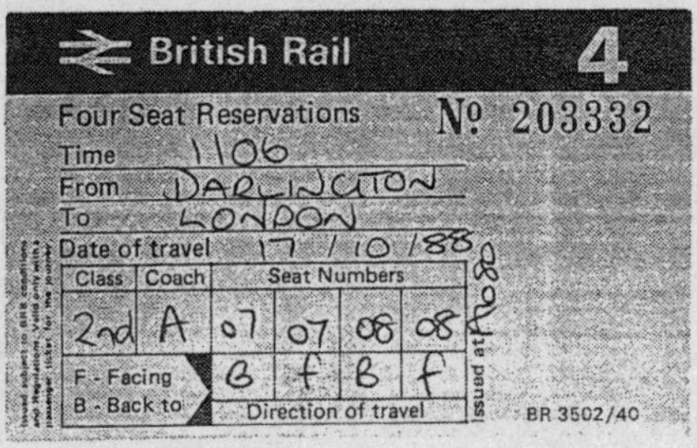
British Rail 4

Four Seat Reservations № 203332

Time 1106

From DARLINGTON

To LONDON

Date of travel 17 / 10 / 88

Class	Coach	Seat Numbers			
2nd	A	07	07	08	08
F - Facing B - Back to		B	f	B	f
		Direction of travel			

Issued at A080

BR 3502/40

Tickets for the train to *Wogan*!

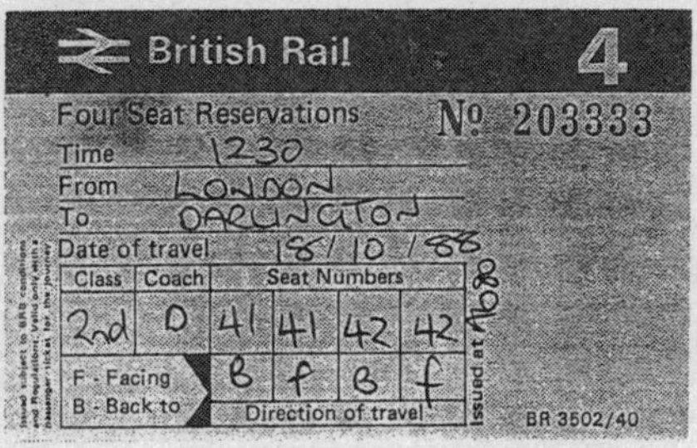
British Rail 4

Four Seat Reservations № 203333

Time 1230

From LONDON

To DARLINGTON

Date of travel 18 / 10 / 88

Class	Coach	Seat Numbers			
2nd	D	41	41	42	42
F - Facing B - Back to		B	f	B	f
		Direction of travel			

Issued at A080

BR 3502/40

It had my name on the door – all for me – I couldn't believe it! Normally when I've been in any shows at home, all the kids get banged into a tiny room, about forty of us, and we are told to just 'shut up', but I had this full dressing room to myself. I thought, I wonder how many famous people have been in here. As I came out I noticed I was right next door to Jean Simmons, the actress. We chatted after the show, she was really nice. We all sat in the dressing room waiting for the call to tell us to go through to Make-up. We were sitting watching *Neighbours* and when it finished the news came on and one of the highlights of the *Six O'Clock News* was *me*!

Terry was very nice, he asked me lots of questions – one of the things he asked me was about my diet and I told him that I ate quite a lot of carob. It was incredible – after the show there was a lady waiting who had brought a box full of carob goodies from the manufacturers, just for me. The power of television! If I ever go back on the TV, I am going to say that bright red sports cars are my favourite!

After the programme we left and went back to the hotel, where there was a lovely surprise for us: Terry had sent a bottle of champagne as a thank you for being on the programme. We decided to keep the champagne for my Five Years Clear party in 1992. (Sadly, Terry couldn't come – but we drank it anyway!) Once again, the next morning our room was filled with journalists and photographers. Some were OK but there was one lady who was a real nutcase – she said to me, 'Are you afraid of dying, Joanne, and what do you think it will be like?' I mean, what sort of question is that? I said, 'Of course I'm afraid of dying, are you looking forward to it?' At that point Mam and Dad said 'Right! That's it! Enough questions – Joanne is concentrating on living and you're asking her questions about dying.' The journalists were all thrown out and our driver took us for a tour around London, before we caught our train back home.

That wasn't to be the end of it, though. When we got to King's Cross the journalists were waiting at the railway station for us again. Some of them even followed us home on the same train. They followed our taxi back to our house and when we got home, there were even more waiting outside our house from local newspapers. I was fed up by this time and I said to them all, 'Look, I'm doing no more pictures and I am going to my friend Claire's house, and her dad's a policeman and if you follow me round there he will arrest you.' So I left them talking to Mam and Dad. They told me later that one man, who was from the *Today* newspaper, said, 'Look, if you really want your work to become a book, send us all away and find yourself a good agent to handle everything for you.' That's what Mam and Dad did. That journalist from the paper – FOUR BROWNIE POINTS!

How things changed after that one appearance on *Wogan*. We were all asked to go back down to London to meet Eric Rowan and Ken Howard from the BBC, to do a children's documentary about cancer. They wanted to chat to us and see if we would agree to the programme being made. While we were down there, we were also invited to a fashion show for the Westminster Children's Hospital. Jeff Banks from *The Clothes Show* was presenting it and he had invited us to stay at his house. Mam, Sarah and I were ever so excited – we had seen him on TV so many times. Dad didn't have a clue who Jeff Banks was, and thought he was probably a footballer. When we arrived at the house we met him and his wife and two children. I said to Jeff, 'Tell Dad which football club you play for.' Jeff looked confused and Dad looked very embarrassed!

The fashion show was good, although some of the clothes were a bit weird and Sarah fell asleep.

The next day we all went to the BBC and had lunch

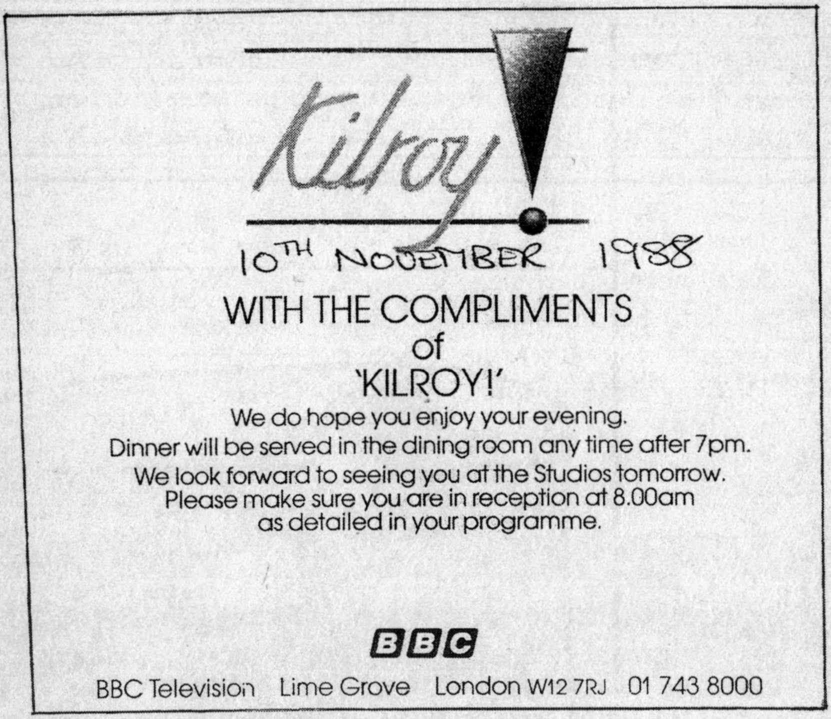

Kilroy!

10TH NOVEMBER 1988

WITH THE COMPLIMENTS
of
'KILROY!'

We do hope you enjoy your evening.
Dinner will be served in the dining room any time after 7pm.
We look forward to seeing you at the Studios tomorrow.
Please make sure you are in reception at 8.00am
as detailed in your programme.

BBC

BBC Television Lime Grove London W12 7RJ 01 743 8000

in the canteen. We met Eric and Ken as arranged and they explained to us about the programme they wanted to make. They asked me if I thought it was a good idea – I mean *seriously*, a programme for half an hour on TV about me! Would *you* turn it down? They said they would like to visit our house in December, film my birthday party, some of my dancing at ballet class and other things.

A couple of days before my birthday Jennifer Kavanagh, the lady who was trying to get my book published, phoned Mam and Dad to tell them that she had found

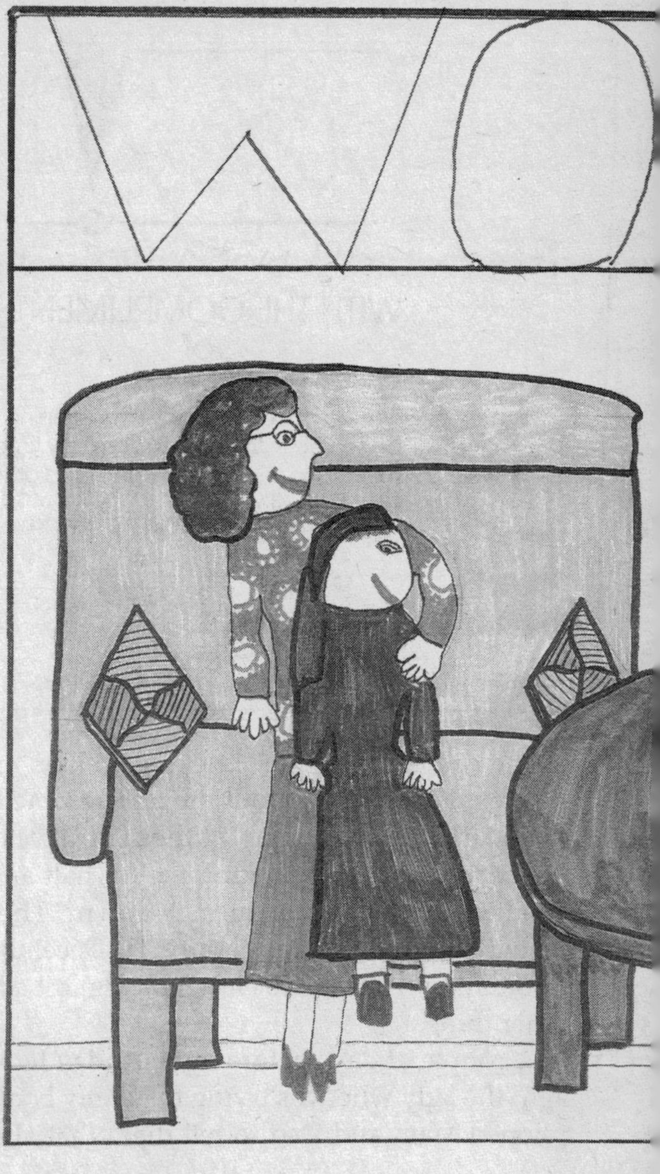
WO

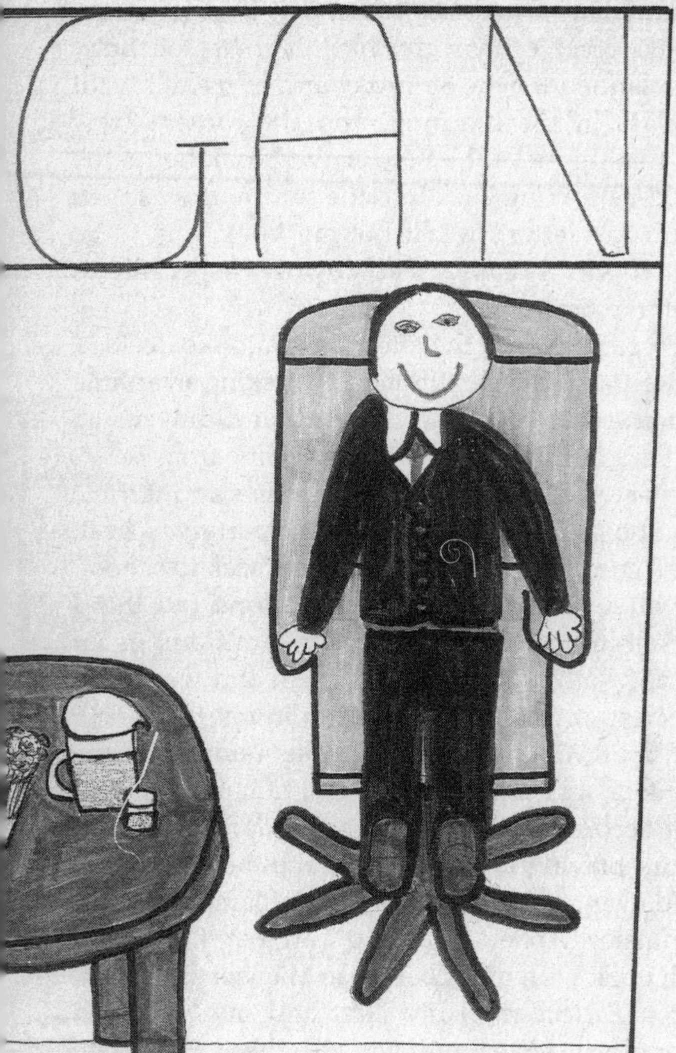
GAN

a publisher. Mam asked her to send it in a letter, so that I would receive it on my birthday. My birthday party was planned for the Saturday and as usual I went to ballet class in the morning, and the camera crew came too, filming me. When we arrived back home the crew filmed us coming back into the house. It was then I picked up my letter, to tell me my book was to be published. It was a really great surprise, especially to find out on my birthday.

My disco party was in the afternoon, and we decided to make the party a little different by asking everyone to come dressed in bad taste clothes that didn't match and were very outrageous, a bit like Aveline from *Bread*. You've never seen so many horrible clothes and terrible colours in one place in your life! But the party was brill. The camera crew went home and I went back to school.

Shortly after returning to school, I found out that I had been selected as one of the Children of Courage for 1988. We all went back to London again and we stayed in the poshest hotel I have ever seen in my life – THE STAKIS ST ERMINS HOTEL. In the middle of the reception area was an enormous Christmas tree, with lights and decorations, and there was a lady at the top of the stairs playing a harp. It was the most beautiful place I had ever seen. There were lots of famous people at Westminster Abbey and you can bet I had my autograph book with me. There was Michael Crawford, Angie from *Eastenders*, Tony Hart and my favourite, Bonnie Langford. Mike Smith was also there. He turned up on crutches (after his helicopter crash) and I think he was every bit as brave as the children. I was asked to read in the Abbey – think of speaking *aloud* in Westminster Abbey, not many people have done that, eh!

After the service we were all going to be introduced to the Duchess of York, Fergie. Mam and Dad had been told the exact procedure when they were to be introduced, to bow or curtsey and say Your Royal Highness. I saw her and I just couldn't hold my tongue. I dashed up and asked her, 'Do you really call the prince "Big Ears"?' She smiled and said, 'I hope you don't mean my prince!' She winked at me and we laughed together. Once again, Mam and Dad were wishing that the floor would open up and swallow them, they were expecting to spend the rest of the week in the Tower. I suppose in the light of recent events she's called her prince a lot worse names than 'Big Ears', but that's none of my business. A couple of hundred years ago, *she* might have ended up in the Tower!

We really enjoyed meeting all those other brave children and their parents and had a great couple of days.

It was almost Christmas again and we were invited to visit the publishers to talk about the book. It wasn't at all like I had imagined, there were books there by loads of famous people and although the staff were friendly and they all seemed to be working very hard, no one really seemed to be making books. Anyway, I suppose they knew what they were doing.

We got hundreds of Christmas cards and letters that year from people all over the place, people we didn't even know. Christmas morning was brill again. We always have the same routine: Sarah and I wake up

Mam and Dad (normally *very early*!), and Dad goes downstairs first, to make sure that Santa has been, or at least that's what he tells us. Once again, Santa had been really kind to us, the living room was covered with presents. We open our presents, have a glass of 'Bucks Fizz' (just a little one!), go to church and then straight on to the children's ward at Middlesbrough General Hospital, where we take a box of chocolates for the nurses. We have done this every year since I came home from hospital. It's just a way of saying thank you for all their help.

After Christmas the BBC camera crew came back to finish filming for *The Lowdown*. One of the things they particularly wanted to film was a thing we do in our house, which involves lighting a candle and sitting round it. You may not understand, so I'll tell you. You know sometimes when there is something you think you want to say, but you feel your Mam and Dad might not understand or be angry with you for saying it? Well, what we do in our house, if it's something that we feel is really important and we want to get it off our chests, we ask for the candle to be lit. We each take turns in speaking and really say what's on our minds; what's either upsetting us or what's pleasing us. While one person speaks no one is allowed to interrupt or answer back. Everyone gets a chance to air their grievances. It gives mams and dads and children a chance to let everyone know exactly how you're feeling, and that you may have problems, some you might not have wanted to talk about, or were afraid of being laughed at. They have to sit there and listen and it gives them a chance to try to understand and maybe to act differently in the future. It really works, and we all feel closer as a family for doing this. Why not try it if you have any problems or are afraid to 'open up'? I'm sure that you will find out a lot about yourself and your family by doing this.

Family Love

Family love is Good, great and fun
Happy times, home and away – but sad times
 will come and arguments too
But love in your family will still be loving you.

The new series of *The Lowdown* was to start at the end of April and mine was to be the first programme in the series. The programme was called 'Brave Heart', after the title of my first book. I'm proud to say that the programme about me went on to win a Royal Award for the best children's documentary on TV. Then again, with such natural talent, beauty and wit, how could it fail!?

My book was published on 4 May and the day before I appeared on *Wogan* for the second time. Terry was his old self but I was disappointed that Michael Jackson was not his musical guest, as I think he's GREAT!!!

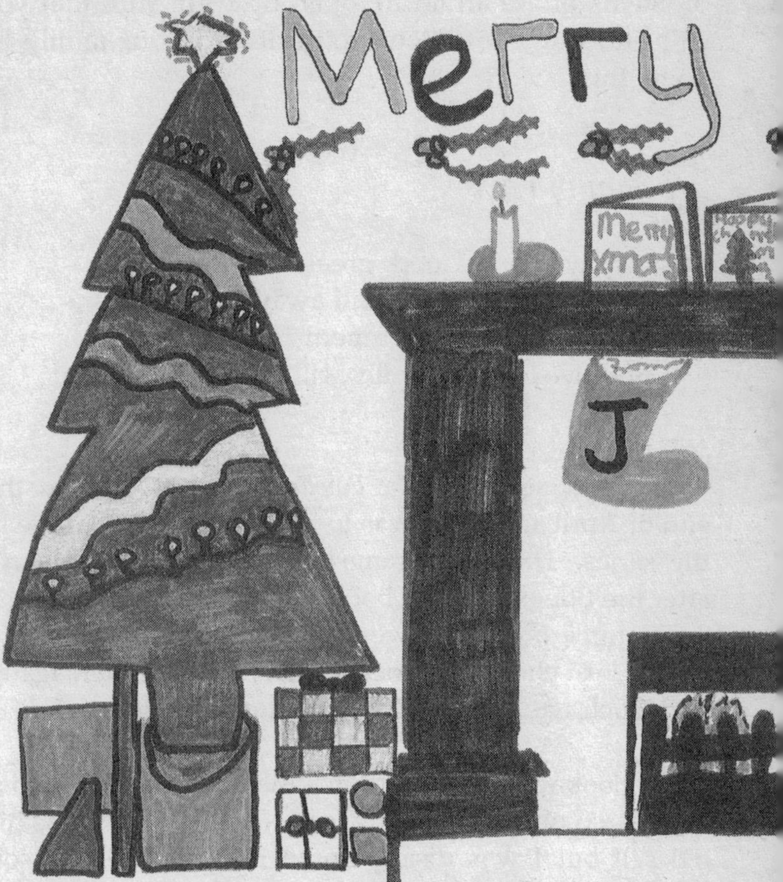
Merry
Merry
xmas
J

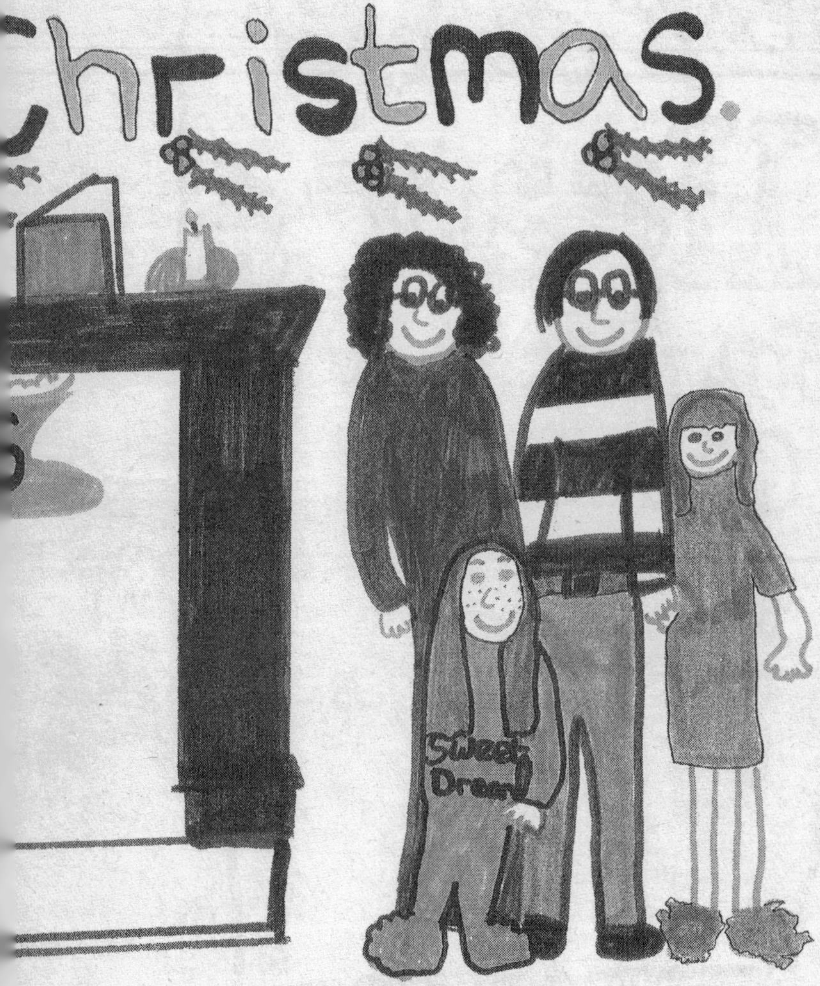
Christmas.
Sweet Dream

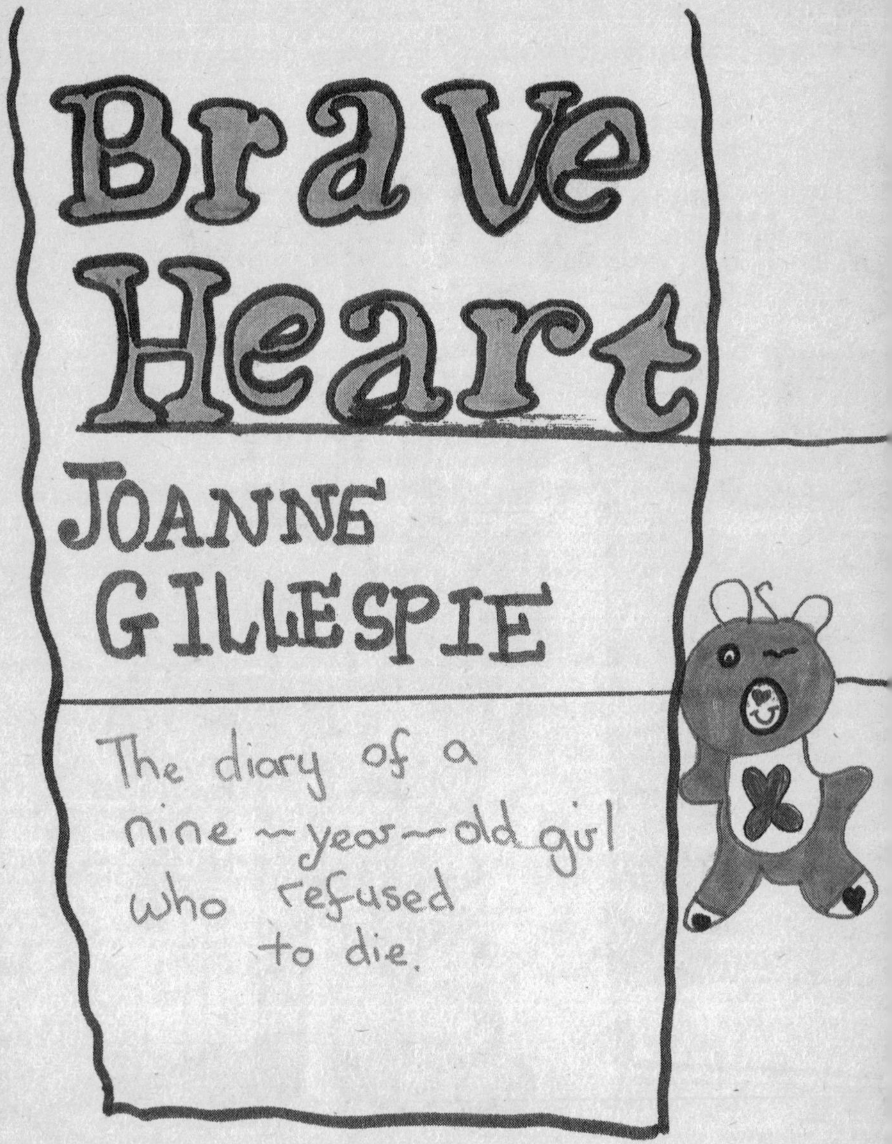

Joanne's first book was published in 1989 and was a bestseller.

Michael Jackson Forever

When I want to annoy my sister
and I want to make really sure
I sing songs by Kylie Minogue
AND CALL HER KYLIE MANURE!!

To help launch the book I did lots of interviews on TV, I was on TV-am and did a workout with Lizzie; I was on radio programmes, did signing sessions in different shops and my favourite bit was on the *Wide Awake Club*. There I met Tommy Boyd, who is one of the nicest people I have met, he was so natural and friendly.

However, I still couldn't understand what all the fuss was about, everybody kept telling me how brave I was but that's not why I wrote the book, I just wrote it to help others.

Brave

Is not a strong man
is not a hero riding
BRAVE is love and peace

In May 1989 I was given an award for Outstanding Human Achievement by the Variety Club of Great Britain. The old autograph book took a real hammering

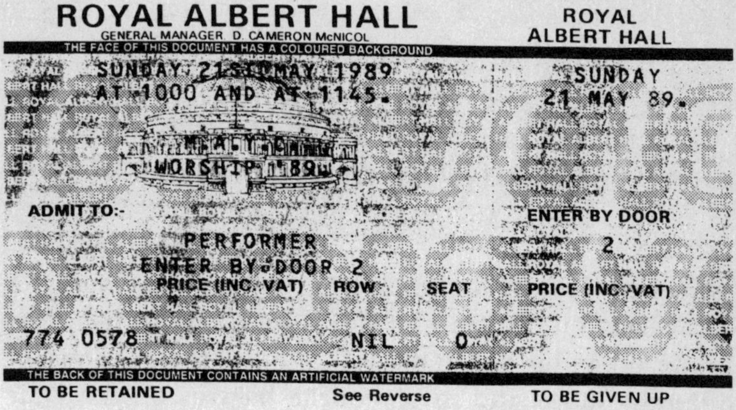
ROYAL ALBERT HALL
GENERAL MANAGER D. CAMERON McNICOL
THE FACE OF THIS DOCUMENT HAS A COLOURED BACKGROUND
SUNDAY 21ST MAY 1989
AT 1000 AND AT 1145.
MAYC
WORSHIP '89
ADMIT TO:-
PERFORMER
ENTER BY DOOR 2
PRICE (INC. VAT) ROW SEAT
774 0578 NIL 0
THE BACK OF THIS DOCUMENT CONTAINS AN ARTIFICIAL WATERMARK
TO BE RETAINED
See Reverse

ROYAL
ALBERT HALL
SUNDAY
21 MAY 89.
ENTER BY DOOR
2
PRICE (INC. VAT)
TO BE GIVEN UP

that night! There were lots of famous people there!

I was beginning to get used to speaking in public by now and on Sunday, 21 May 1989, I was invited to speak at the MAYC weekend, at the Royal Albert Hall in London. The MAYC is the Methodist Association of Youth Clubs and every year thousands and thousands of young people from churches all over the country meet together to worship, and I was asked to speak to them. I was asked to have something ready to say, and when it was my turn on stage, I went out and said:

> 'Hi, I'm Joanne, I want to tell you about God and the help He has given me, and that whatever may go wrong, never doubt that He is there. You see about three years ago, I had my first of two operations to remove a brain tumour, after that I had a stroke and a course of radiotherapy and all my hair fell out. Sometimes I felt really down, but I knew I would get better because both me and

God were fighting it. Sometimes, I would think "Why me?" but then I would realize that God didn't give me cancer and He doesn't give us any other diseases either, but He does try to get us through and it is important that we help ourselves as well. So remember to trust in God, even though some days it may feel like God is not helping you, those are the days when He is trusting you. Don't think it will always be easy though, because it can be very hard. Don't give up your battle, because it's when things seem hardest that you might be near to winning. So don't be scared. *I have put all my faith in God and I know that cancer will never kill me, if I die it will be because God wants me*. But He doesn't want me just yet. The doctors are surprised I'm still here and some days I still get funny feelings in my fingers, but I'm still fighting and still praying, so keep on fighting when you're hardest hit – it's when things seem worse that you mustn't quit.'

As I said, the place was full of teenagers and for almost two minutes they gave me a standing ovation. As everyone left and we were escorted through to a back room, one of the men who organized the event said he was really impressed by what I'd said, and after I returned home I received some letters from other people who had been there and had heard me, saying how much it had helped them.

Well, things seemed to slow down after that. For a couple of weeks I had been really famous, my book sold well which meant I could give money to our local hospital for new equipment and also to give some money to our church, to buy some new bibles.

FIGHTERS

Fighters are people that get hit on the chin

Fighters are people that do like to win

Fighters are people with dreams in their heads

Fighters are people that get up from their beds

Fighters are people that give it a try

Fighters are people that know when to cry

Fighters are people that although they fall,

they pick themselves up and don't cry at all

So give it a try, stick out your chin

Roll up your sleeves and then GET STUCK IN!

Also, just as important, it gave parents and children contact with someone who had been through these troubles. I had often heard Mam and Dad say that people thought they knew how they felt, but they didn't really, and if mams and dads felt like that, imagine how frightened children would be.

We received lots of letters and Mam would spend hours on the telephone just listening to other mothers whose children were in a similar situation. I had trouble writing, as my right hand wasn't very good and I was teaching myself to write left-handed, and I couldn't possibly answer all the people who had asked me to write. So we started making cassettes. I made a master-tape and told the children everything I had done and what they could do to help themselves and Mam would just send copies out whenever we received a letter. Sometimes we would travel to the hospital, as people would contact us and ask us to visit a particular family who had just found out that their child had cancer. We would go to try to encourage them to stay cheerful and never give up. I would tell them that you can get better, I'm getting better and I'm going to stay better – it's up to you, but you've got to try.

I spent my last few weeks at junior school, where I had been very happy – the teachers and the headmistress, Mrs Carnell, had always been very nice to me. When the term finished, I spent six weeks very excited and nervous at the same time, wondering what senior school would be like. WAS I IN FOR A SHOCK!

Some of the kids at the new school were grown ups! They were huge! But some who, just like me, had started that day and had come from other schools around the area, felt very small and insignificant.

Some were not very nice, and I had never come across children like them. They had seen me on TV and in newspapers, they had seen me meeting famous people, and they seemed to be jealous – jealous of the people I had met and things I had done. Try as I would, there was no way I could win them over. It seems they just didn't like me. I felt very alone and very sad that I had left my junior school, where everyone was a friend and understood me. I was soon to learn just to be myself and if people didn't like me then that was just tough.

<u>DON'T</u>

Don't say Can't
Don't say Don't
Don't say Never
Don't say Wont

Don't just stand there
Don't do that
Don't say nothing
Don't back chat

Don't watch tele
Don't eat those
Don't bite your fingers
Don't pick your nose

Don't be late
Don't get wet
Don't be lazy
Don't go yet

Don't start crying
Don't just grin
Don't get poorly
<u>DON'T GIVE IN</u>

First Year at Senior School
or
Lines, Lines and *More* Lines

I was really nervous when I first started senior school. We had been told all the rules of the school – such as, *You must be on time for classes, if you are late, you could get a detention, or even lines*. This proved a bit awkward for me. In junior school we stayed at the same desk, but in senior school we could be at one end of the school for one lesson and right down the other end for the next. We have to carry our books and PE equipment with us. Some days, by two o'clock, I felt totally knackered! This moving from class to class caused a further problem for me – Mam and Dad had always told me the important thing was to get there, never mind about being late. I haven't got very good balance and it seems whenever I'm pushed or stumble, because I can't get my hands out to save myself, I always fall down on my bad hand and either sprain or break my wrist, and so because I'm a bit slow, other people tend not to want to walk with me. Some days I just manage to get into the class in time, otherwise I would be writing two pages of the old:

I MUST LEARN TO GET HERE ON TIME, IT IS AN IMPORTANT PART OF MY GROWING UP!
I MUST LEARN TO GET HERE ON TIME, IT IS AN IMPORTANT PART OF MY GROWING UP!
I MUST LEARN TO GET HERE ON TIME, IT IS AN IMPORTANT PART OF MY GROWING UP!
I MUST LEARN TO GET HERE ON TIME, IT IS AN IMPORTANT PART OF MY GROWING UP!
I MUST LEARN TO GET HERE ON TIME, IT IS AN IMPORTANT PART OF MY GROWING UP!

There were some things I was told I must not do. Mrs Johnson, my physiotherapist, had already visited the school and told them I must not play hockey, in case I was hit on the head with a stick, and I must not climb ropes or wall bars as obviously, with only one good hand, I could easily fall and, again, bump my head. Somersaults and exercises like that used to make me feel quite sick and dizzy so I wasn't to do those, either. Lots of the kids used to say I was really lucky not having to do these things, but before my operations I used to love PE and games: I used to play tennis and golf, I even used to go to gymnastics at a local sports hall. Because they didn't like it and had to do it, they thought I was lucky – SOME LUCK, EH? I mean if I was really lucky, Mrs Johnson would have stopped me from doing cross-country which I hate, but she didn't! Still, if I *did* do PE, etc, the effects would stop me from enjoying what I *can* do. All right, so I can't catch a ball very well now and I might not be a very good shot at netball or games like that, but I still enjoy doing them.

I suppose I'm like a bird with one wing, sad I can't fly but glad I can sing!

I've chatted with some famous people,
and I've often been seen on TV
Some people look on in envy,
I wish they could see the real me.
The Newspapers call me 'Kid Courage'
and tell me I've got what it takes,
The girl who fought back against cancer,
But worries when she gets headaches.

Some kids say 'I'm willing to swop you',
All those brilliant things that you do
They forget that having cancer's unpleasant
and everyone doesn't pull through.
They forget about fear and sickness,
and they don't know a thing about pain
and recovering is not always easy
when you're minus a bit of your brain!

A few of them seem really jealous,
and say things that aren't nice at all
Baldy, or ugly or fatty
She's useless, she can't catch a ball
Then the black looks all turn into punches
and the stories turn into lies
It seems, for winning my fight against cancer,
Being disliked is my prize.

Well, I guess that I must just be different,
and I might as well go my own way,
I've given up all I intend to,
They simply don't want me to play
No bicycle, hockey or skating,
and never will I dance the Swan,
Fingers that once were so nimble,
Like my dreams, all the feelings have gone.

So remember when you think that I'm lucky,
That they haven't been easy these years
Losing the things I once dreamed of
and watching my parents hide tears,
So don't think that I'm all goody, goody,
and think that I never go wrong,
For if God wanted me for an angel
He'd not have let me live quite so long!

Apart from PE, the only real problems I had were (1) the amount of homework I got, which came as a shock to everybody who started in the first year and (2) one particular teacher, who seemed to enjoy nothing better than standing me up in front of the rest of the class and making a total prat out of me. It got to the point that I was so afraid of this teacher, it was bringing spasms on in my hand. I didn't want the others in my class to think I couldn't handle it and I knew that if I told my mam or dad, they would have come to the school to sort it out. I knew this meant that some would scoff at me and say sarcastically, 'Do your parents fight all your battles for you . . . ?' but I wish I'd told them earlier. I didn't feel I could ask for help, and because of my hand I couldn't write as fast as the others: I seemed to be getting further and further behind. I wanted so much to be just like the others. They seemed to say all kinds of things to the teachers and get away with it; when I spoke out, I was told not to be cheeky, just because I had been on television, but if I didn't say anything, the kids would say I must be a goody-two-shoes, a proper teacher's pet!

One day I just couldn't take any more, I broke down in front of my mam and dad and told them that I was just so terrified of this teacher. They were really understanding, although they were a bit annoyed I had taken so long to tell them and they went straight to school to see the headmaster. The headmaster told them he would have words with the teacher and try to sort the whole thing out. He also thought the teacher concerned didn't fully understand my situation and assumed my slow work was down to my being lazy.

I don't know if the headmaster did actually speak to the teacher or not. If he did, all that happened was that things got worse. One day I was talking to my PE teacher. While we were chatting, I had quite a painful spasm in my hand.

She had never seen this happen before, and now understood why I couldn't do most of the PE exercises. My next lesson was with the teacher I was having problems with. My spasms can be made worse if I get nervous or over-excited. I was getting worried that I would get lines for being late and this made my spasms stronger. My PE teacher said I must not go until the spasms had stopped. It was a vicious circle – I was told not to worry and to tell my next teacher what had happened. That was a waste of time as I was given the lines anyway and told that I knew the rules and no excuses would be accepted!

My dad thought I must have been cheeky to one of the teachers, called me a 'wally' and said it served me right, but when I told him why I had got the lines, he nearly blew a fuse! He took the sheet off me and wrote across the bottom:

> 'JOANNE WILL NOT BE DOING THESE LINES, AND I WILL BE AT SCHOOL TOMORROW TO SORT IT OUT.'

The next day I handed my lines in – I was sort of relieved and afraid at the same time. I could tell by their faces that people were not amused by what Dad had written. When Mam and Dad got to the school, the headmaster said to them, 'Well, it's school policy to give children lines.' I think he was surprised because they agreed with him. But when they told him the events that had caused the lines to be given, he agreed that in those circumstances the lines shouldn't have been given to me. Dad then went on to say that he felt giving me a set number of lines to do was unfair because it took me so long to write them and what he and the headmaster agreed was, if ever this was the case in future, then I would do twenty or thirty minutes, so that the punishment wasn't too unfair. I mean, if I'd only had one leg, they wouldn't have expected me to run twice round the rugby pitch like everyone else, would they?

During the couple of weeks that followed, it seemed obvious that something had been said to the teacher. She wasn't any nicer to me, nor any more helpful either, though I must admit this was partially my fault because I was still too afraid to ask for help. But it was obvious now that I wasn't being singled out quite so much or humiliated any more.

I have had lines to do a couple of times since then, but this is mainly my dad's fault! I mean, he does have a car, but he makes me walk to school every day, unless it's absolutely pouring down! Sometimes, I hang about and plead, 'Please, please give me a lift!' But it doesn't work and of course I can end up being late for school – and then I hear the same words as soon as I walk in: I MUST LEARN TO BE PUNCTUAL – IT IS AN IMPORTANT PART OF MY GROWING UP. The funny thing is, though, on the few occasions when I have had lines to do, I always feel I have let myself and my parents down in some way, but they just smile and tell me not to worry and that it's OK, it happens to everybody. I realize now that my parents didn't go to the school because I had lines at all, they went there because they thought I was being unfairly treated.

Towards the end of the first term, the school had an open night for parents of first-year children. Mam and Dad were quite pleased as all the teachers they spoke to agreed that, although I might never be the Brain of

Britain, I tried my very best and did the best I could under the circumstances. Sure, my writing was slow, but it was improving as were other things that people take for granted, like drawing a straight line with the ruler, and the school had agreed to let me start using my dictation machine so that I could put homework on to it, or any notes that were needed, to save me time from writing. This was great and saved me loads of time, though, obviously, there were some people who said, 'It's not fair, *we* can't use one of those.'

I thought at the start of the new term things would get better – but it wasn't to be. Once again my teacher made me look so foolish that I started off a spasm. The spasm got stronger and stronger and by the time I had reached the next lesson – Mrs Garside, who took me for Drama – I was in such a state that she said I had better go home. My spasms normally only run for a few minutes, and then they pass, but this was so strong that it lasted the whole day at school. My arm felt almost dead and I was getting a strange twitching feeling in my mouth. I had only really had this feeling once before, and this was the day I had a stroke. Mam and Dad tried to relax me, but no matter what they did, I just didn't seem able to stop the spasm from running down my arm, and my lip was becoming more and more numb. They decided the best thing they could do was to get me to Mr Nath and hope he would be able to have a look at me. He did manage to get to see me and he confirmed what my mam and dad had said, that I must learn not to let people upset me, not to get annoyed and to come to terms with these spasms otherwise I would be suffering from them for ever. I don't know if it was because I had the security of having Mam, Dad and Sarah beside me and all the other doctors and nurses in the hospital, but I did start to feel a little easier.

Mr Nath said, 'Look, Joanne, you are about due for a brain scan, so I think we should have one done while you're here.' I thought, 'Oh, yes, great, inject my arm with blue dye, this is going to make me feel much better!' I don't really like having the brain scan, but I knew I had to have one sooner or later, and I was there, so I decided to get it over and done with. The brain scan from my position was boring as usual and, if it hadn't been for my mam being there, I think I would have been really fed up. Mam had to wear a special lead jacket – she really suits lead, my mam! – this was to make sure she wasn't affected by the x-rays from the machine. The scan was completed and we went back to Mr Nath's office. He walked in with the x-rays and, as I have said, I may not be the brightest person in the world but I am also not the silliest either and I could tell straightaway something was wrong.

He put the x-rays on a screen that lit up on the wall and showed my mam and dad pictures of my brain. My brain with a tumour on it, the size of a plum! The tumour had come back. Although they weren't crying, I could see Mam and Dad were unable to speak. An excuse was made and Mr Nath's secretary took me and Sarah out of the room so he could have a chat with Mam and Dad. He knew they had always told me the truth and felt this was not the time to start doing

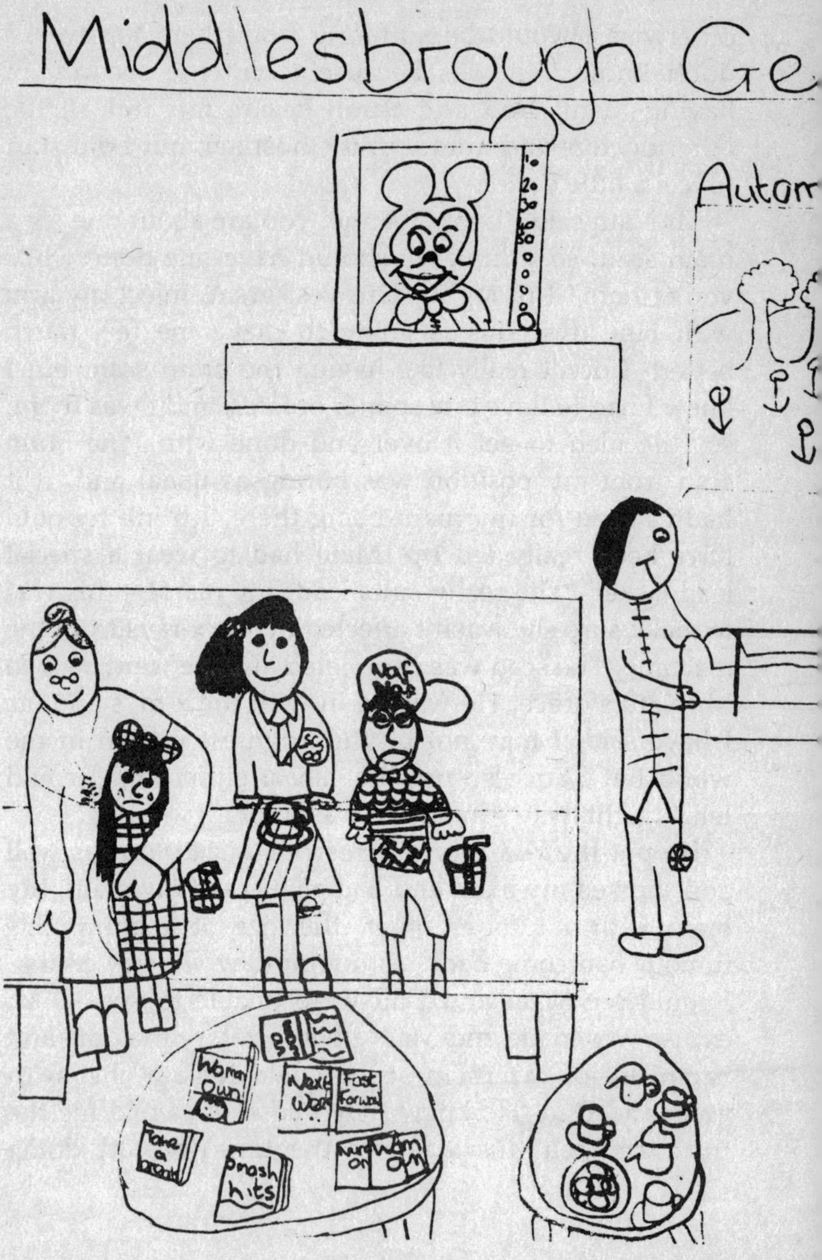
Middlesbrough Ge
Autom
Naf Naf
Woman Own
Next Week
Fast Forwa
Take a break
Smash hits
Wom Own

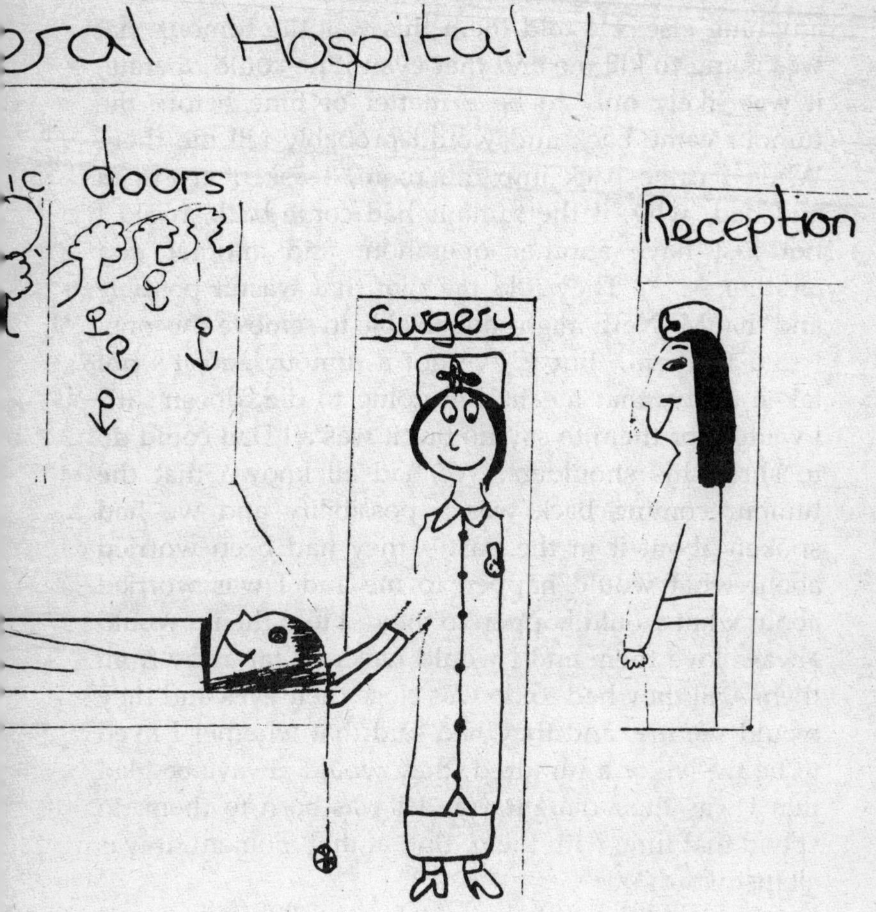

Hospital
doors
Reception
Sugery

anything else. He told them this was the tumour that was going to kill me and that even if he could operate, it was likely only to be a matter of time before the tumour came back and would probably kill me then. When I came back into the room, I asked my mam and dad, why, if the tumour had come back, could I not just have another operation, and another and another . . . ? They told me that that wasn't possible and that Mr Nath might not be able to remove this one. I said to them, 'But if I've got a tumour and it's not taken away, that means I'm going to die, doesn't it?' I waited for them to say no but it was all Dad could do to shrug his shoulders. We had all known that the tumour coming back was a possibility and we had spoken about it in the past – they had been worried about what would happen to me and I was worried about what would happen to them. I told them I would always love them and I would never be far away from them – all they had to do was close their eyes and they would see me, and they had said that whether I lived to be twelve or a hundred, they would always be glad that I was their daughter and I was born to them, to spend that time with them. But, at that moment, it was all just words.

As we sat there, I thought to myself, 'Well this is great, I only came in because I had a spasm and now I find I've got a brain tumour.' I sat for a bit longer and I thought to myself, 'Well, I don't feel like I've got a brain tumour.' Mam said, 'I wonder when Mr Nath will get the appointment for us in London,' and I told them, 'Look, we should stop worrying until we've had the result of the scan: we should be more positive.' We went home and waited for our appointment.

Memo from Dad

It always seems that when the chips are down, the best comes out of Joanne.

We had taken her to hospital, telling her to be more confident and stop letting people upset her, to try to be in control of these spasms. We left a few hours later, after being told our daughter was dying, and yet it was her who turned the tables on us again. We left that hospital with a false confidence, but at least it was some sort of confidence. This was given to us by Joanne – had it been left to us, we would just have sat there crying, but she wanted to continue to fight and if Joanne wanted to continue the fight, Mam and Dad would help her.

Mr Nath had wanted a special scan, which was only available in London, and he had made the arrangements for us to travel down. He was due to go on holiday and had asked if we could bring the scan results back with us from London, and take them directly to his office, so he could compare them with the scan taken at Middlesbrough General, in order to make necessary arrangements to perform surgery on his return from holiday.

SOARING THROUGH THE AIR

Is it a bird?

Is it a plane?

NO its a hurtling golf ball

Zooming

Wooshing

There goes another one

As fast as a missile

As quick as a cheetah

I hit one myself.........but it only went a metre

Just missed a bunker

Oops into the woods

Well.......Just have to get lessons

Just before we went to London, two things happened; one, Dave Martin from MAYC (Methodist Association of Youth Clubs) had written to Mam and Dad just to ask how I was. Mam had written back, telling them exactly what the situation was and asking if they would all pray for me. Secondly, Miss Hutchinson, who used to be my teacher at junior school, had told Mam and Dad about a preacher who was coming to her church, called Derek Prince. He was coming from America and was quite a well-known healer. They decided to take me to the church to see him.

Halfway through the service Mr Prince asked if anyone who needed healing would go to the front of the church with a supporter. Dad and I went to the front and, as we stood there with other people, he made his way along. Dad stood behind me; eventually Mr Prince stood in front of me and put his hands on my head. I don't really know what happened next, my legs just crumbled, it was as if I had been hit in the face. Dad grabbed me before I hit the floor. I could hear Dad saying, 'What have you done?' and Mr Prince saying, 'It's OK, don't worry, she'll be all right.' A chair was brought for me to sit on and Dad still stood behind me to stop me from falling from the chair. I was in a sort of half-asleep, half-awake state; I could hear everything that was being said, and what was going on, but it just felt so comfortable, I didn't want to wake up. I stayed on that chair for about twenty minutes according to Dad, and when I woke up I knew exactly what had been said. Dad said *I* had been chatting away all the time, although I wasn't aware of that. We went back and sat with Mam and Sarah and I felt really fine. As we sat there, Mr Prince came back to me and in front of all the congregation, said, 'I want everyone here to pray for this girl, she has been very ill.' We had been to see healers before, but nothing like that had ever happened. My dad has said several times since that if he had seen that with anyone else he would have thought it was fixed, a put-up job, but we had no idea what was going to happen, and with me being already 'out' I had no idea that the same thing happened to other people after me.

SPRING

Spring is the day when life arrives
The flowers blossom before your very eyes
The grass is green, the lambs are born
Everything fresh on this new spring morn
The chicks in their nets sing a sweet song
Springs when everythings right - not wrong
Spring - everyone loves that day
Nobody can take spring away

Memo from Dad

We set off for London the next day. Before Joanne and Kathy could go into the room where the scan was, they were asked if they had a pacemaker or anything metal with batteries with them. They had to take their watches off and any jewellery. Joanne had the scan and the x-rays were given to us in a sealed envelope, which we brought straight back up to the North East and gave to Mr Nath the very next day. Once again, he put the x-rays on the screen. He looked at them and said, 'Oh, this is wrong, you've been given the wrong scan.' He put up the original ones that he had taken earlier in Middlesbrough and showed us the tumour. He compared them with the new ones and said, 'There is nothing there! There must be some sort of mistake. Certainly, there is some damage, but this isn't Joanne's.' He told us he would contact London and get a detailed report as to what exactly the scans were saying. He said he would get back in touch with us later on that day and let us know what was happening. We left the hospital excited and confused. The report from the MRI (Magnetic Resonance Imaging) came through. It said that although there was some residual damage to Joanne's brain from previous surgery, there was no sign of any recurrence of the tumour at all.

We were ecstatic! But Mr Nath still couldn't go along with it and he told us he would send the file and reports to a professor he had studied under in Scotland for a second opinion. Whatever *he* said, Mr Nath would go along with. The professor in Scotland wrote back after studying the reports and said that he tended to go along with the MRI scan. Mr Nath was delighted to be proved wrong, although he still couldn't understand it. Something had happened, something very strange and something very powerful. We all knew what had happened to the tumour – although we can't prove it, we are positive that God worked through Mr Prince that night and made Joanne well!

I was kept off school for another few days. Eventually, I went back with my mam and dad and we saw the headmaster. We told him exactly what had happened. I suppose, in a strange way, it was a good thing – that teacher may well have caused the spasms to come on that day, so it was agreed I should change class. AND I DID. There wasn't really much more that happened that term – well, unless you include having a local charity, 'Brave Hearts of the North East', named after my book, and being on stage with Dire Straits. If you want to know more about that – read on! I've got loads of homework to do, and *Neighbours* will be on TV soon, and I do get fed up after a while – SEE YOU LATER!

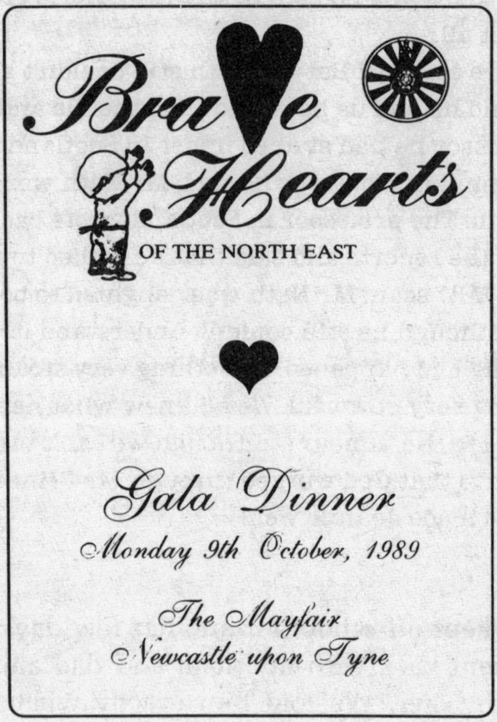
Brave Hearts
OF THE NORTH EAST
Gala Dinner
Monday 9th October, 1989
The Mayfair
Newcastle upon Tyne

Thank You for Being a Friend

HELLO AGAIN! Right, as I've said, I won an award for 'Outstanding Human Achievement' from the Variety Club of Great Britain. It was a really lovely night, I've never seen my mam and dad look so tidy before. Mam always looks smart in nice dresses but my dad was wearing a 'dickie bow' and a black suit! Anyway, as the night went on I was given my award and I had to make a speech. When I had finished speaking, the people all stood up and gave me a round of applause. Afterwards, I found out that there were some people from the Hexham Round Table and some people from Newcastle Breweries and they thought that it would be a good idea if a charity was launched for other children in the North East who had been particularly brave in illness, by helping others or by overcoming some obstacle. They asked if they could call the charity after my book *Brave Heart*. They would hope to send some children on a special holiday or, if travelling was impossible, to buy them something they had always wanted, like a computer or, in some cases, maybe an electronic wheelchair to make life easier.

I was really pleased to be asked to help, and to have the charity named after my book was a real honour. On

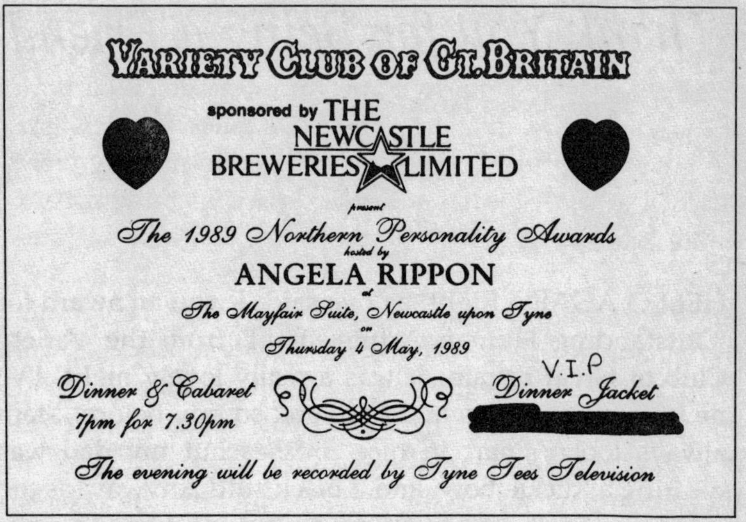

VARIETY CLUB OF GT. BRITAIN

sponsored by THE NEWCASTLE BREWERIES LIMITED

present

The 1989 Northern Personality Awards

hosted by

ANGELA RIPPON

at

The Mayfair Suite, Newcastle upon Tyne

on

Thursday 4 May, 1989

Dinner & Cabaret
7pm for 7.30pm

V.I.P
Dinner Jacket
[redacted]

The evening will be recorded by Tyne Tees Television

the night of the launch of the charity, we all travelled to Newcastle, and there were some lovely people in the audience. Lots were businessmen who were making donations for raffles, etc, to raise money towards the fund. Some people gave flights to America, hotels had 'weekends for two' and Dire Straits gave a framed golden disc of one of their records to be put up for auction.

When it was time to draw the numbers for the raffle, Sarah was asked to draw one and she pulled out her own ticket and won a set of crystal glasses for Mam and Dad! They were over the moon! There was a group, a singer and a comedian (sorry, it wasn't a comedian, it was Frank Carson!) and then after a while the compère said, 'And now, we are delighted to introduce Dire Straits, live on stage!' The audience almost fell off their seats! I fought my way through to the front and stood there watching, sort of half dancing, and one of the group was asking me to come up on stage. Well, you know me, I don't have to be asked twice – quick as a flash I was up there, dancing with them as they were playing. It was great – afterwards we met them back stage and they gave us both copies of their LP and signed them for Sarah and me. We still have them.

My first year at senior school would soon be coming to an end, we had done all the normal end-of-term things, and after six glorious weeks of holidays, I would be going back. But not as a first year, this time I would be in the second year and a little bit more confident of the things I would be doing. Problem was, lots of the lads seemed to have got more confident too. They really fancied themselves and thought all the girls would be falling over themselves to get at them.

School

At school, some of the boys treat me like a fool
It's always the other girls that they say are cool,
But I don't care
Let them stare or pull my hair
because I'm alive
I've got Disco and Jive
I've got the best
Family and Friends
and as for the rest –
Well, who needs boys?

They would stand there, with their hair slicked back, saying things like, 'Come on, baby, you know you want me!' Mam said, 'Boys can be funny at that age,' but they didn't seem funny to me. To be honest, despite the effort that most of them were making to be macho and sexy, most of them could easily be mistaken for dog food! Now I'm not saying I'm perfect (although I am, I'm not saying it!), I do believe us girls deserve a little bit better than that.

HIM

I used to think he was smashing

The best boy in our school

Now hes a total divvy

A dimwit, a wally, a fool

And anyway, who needs boyfriends - not me

He can go boil his head!

He's spotty, and smelly and awful

I'd rather cuddle my ted

His skin's like a boxfull of Brillo

and his face is a terrible mess

And if he dare ask me to the school disco

I THINK THAT I WOULD TELL HIM 'YES'

It was during the second year at school that one of the saddest things happened to me. I suddenly realized that I was unable to carry on with my ballet dancing. I simply could not hold my balance once I got into senior grade. My leg just wasn't strong enough and my right arm was too weak. I have to do everything *100 per cent*, and found it very hard not to be able to do the things I had always taken for granted. It was very upsetting at first to realize that I would never be a famous dancer. It had always been my ambition to be the best, to dance in *Swan Lake*, and it came as quite a shock to realize that this would never be. Deep down, I had known for a while that I was starting to fall behind in class, but I kept trying and coming home each week very, very upset. After a talk with Mam and Dad, I had to accept that it was time to leave my lovely ballet. I still enjoy watching it and will travel anywhere to see ballet. My mam told me a saying: 'Where one door closes, another one opens,' and within a couple of weeks of leaving dancing class, there was a telephone call from our local drama group. My name had been on the waiting list for a few years, as I am also very interested in drama, and I had finally reached the top of the list!

The Journey

We're all on a journey,
A journey of hope
There's no time to worry
or to sit down and mope.

We have to be certain
that we will win
if we just keep on fighting
and remember to grin.

I have picked up quite a few tips since starting, which has helped in our local Church Pantomime. This year the whole family was involved. We were performing *Aladdin* – I was the genie, Dad was Widow Twanky, Mam was in the chorus and Sarah was a mummy, dressed from head to toe in bandages. Obviously, because of her size, she had to be a 'Mini-Mummy' . . . Dad said she should have had two cans of Coke beside her, so that people would realize she was 'TWO TIN CARMEN!' (HA HA!)

Anyway, as I've said, I was the genie and so I had to act very superior and far too important to talk to mere mortals. I had to keep a straight face all the time. This proved to be a bit too hard one night – you see, being a genie, I turned my dad, who was a dame, into a mermaid. He told me he wanted his legs back and with a flash and a wave of my hands, the magic spell was said and Dad turned back into Widow Twanky. At that point he was supposed to wave his legs up in the air from behind a bath in which he was sitting. So, lying on his back, Dad kicked his legs about in the air – of course all of the cast could see my dad from the sidelines, and he had forgotten to put his pantomime knickers on! He looked ever so cute in his red underpants and tights! Everyone burst out laughing and it was really hard remembering our lines. It's always sad on the last night of a pantomime, everyone has put so much effort in to make the show a success, that you don't really want it to finish, especially when people have been enjoying themselves and give you a round of applause and cheers. There's always the next year to look forward to though.

When Mam sent the Christmas cards off last year, she put a note in each one, reminding everyone that 1992 would be the year of my 'Thank you for being a friend party' and that she would write back nearer the time with exact dates. We had the invitations printed and towards the end of February we started preparing the

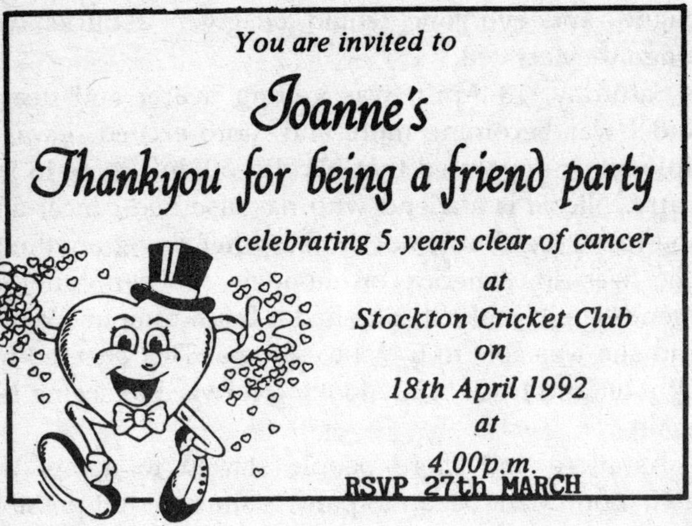
You are invited to

Joanne's

Thankyou for being a friend party

celebrating 5 years clear of cancer

at

Stockton Cricket Club

on

18th April 1992

at

4.00p.m.

RSVP 27th MARCH

final list of guests to invite. Sadly, many were unable to come, as it was held on Easter Saturday, but I have great memories of the times I spent with them over the past five years, and they will never be far away from my thoughts, even though they couldn't make it.

As we got into March and people started replying, it was time to sit down and think about catering. Friends of ours from church run a small catering company called Posh Nosh and they said they would do it for us. I had to choose a menu. I just wanted things that could be picked up easily and eaten quickly, so that people wouldn't be kept off the dance floor! I wanted them to have a really good time. I had a really brilliant cake made by Mam's friend Norma – it was pink and white icing, in the shape of a heart (my favourite shape!) and had written on it 'THANK YOU FOR BEING A FRIEND'. Dad had been saving up to buy some champagne, and everyone would be given a Bucks Fizz when they arrived.

Saturday, 18 April, was getting nearer and nearer and I was becoming more and more excited. I was a little bit disappointed that Nicola couldn't come to my party. Nicola is a friend who has also had cancer and she lost a leg, but it doesn't stop her doing anything. She was in America on holiday. Colleen, another friend, could make it. She had a brain tumour like me and she was able to travel to see me. That cheered me up a bit and I was really looking forward to seeing her again.

As more and more people started to accept the invitation, Mam began to panic – she couldn't possibly have everyone coming with the house in such a state. IT WOULD JUST HAVE TO BE DECORATED! Well, I did say that we call her the Tidy Police! This really chuffed Dad and he set to decorating the hall with a cheery smile on his face, just like a man who knows he's headed for certain death. Of course with this ploy working, Mam decided there were lots of other jobs that needed doing around the house – the sad thing was that, the more jobs there were to be done, Dad started giving me and Sarah more things to do too! I was so fed up by this stage with all the cleaning that was going on, that when I was asked to write a poem called 'My Room' for our church Eisteddfod, I entered one I had already written about my room being attacked by the Tidy Police and it won first prize! Thanks Mam for the inspiration – and the perspiration!

My Room

My room is hopeless, I can't find a thing
I can't find my books, there's no clothes in the bin
No clothes on the bed, or the chair, or the floor
no socks on my computer, no coat on the door,
no pens on my desk. A mess that took hours –
is polished and sparkling and smelling of flowers
Not one bit of rubbish, not one little piece
My room's been attacked by the TIDY POLICE!

P.S. That's what we call Mam, when she gets the cleaning bug!

Well, the Easter holidays finally arrived. I set to doing all my homework, getting it finished so that I could have as much time as possible to myself to prepare for the party, and on Good Friday Colleen arrived to spend the night with us ready for the party. We were also going to celebrate Dad's fortieth birthday that weekend. Yes, my dad is forty – he has finally had to admit to the fact that he is over the hill!

Everyone was very busy and on the Saturday morning the final preparations were being made. Some friends of ours, Anne and Les, had offered to help by picking any guests up who needed lifts. One of the special guests was Jeff Banks, the clothes designer; he came directly from Peru. He met his wife at Heathrow and they flew together straight to Teesside. He had spent thirty-six hours travelling to get to my party and I was really thrilled that he had taken so much time and trouble to be with me – it meant so much. He had promised three years earlier to make it, but so had a lot of other people, and I don't think they had to make quite so much effort as he did. Another special guest was Tommy Boyd from Children's ITV. He had interviewed me three years earlier on the *Wide Awake Club* and I had got on really well with him. He also kept his promise to come and he brought his dad and his son Jack. Our local TV personalities came too, some reporters from our local newspaper, Jennifer Kavanagh (my agent!) who helped me to get my first book published as well as this one, Keith Proud from our local radio station and his wife, two of our very special friends, all my family, aunties and uncles, my two

Nanas, my best friends from school, my school teacher and friends from church, not forgetting Mr Nath, who has looked after me for so long, and his new wife. Some of the nurses from Ward 9 also came.

IT WAS A VERY SPECIAL DAY, WITH VERY SPECIAL PEOPLE AROUND ME. It was so lovely that I couldn't stop myself from shedding a few tears, I was so overcome by the whole thing. I HAD REALLY MADE IT! The party was a way of saying thank you to all those wonderful people who had helped and encouraged me to stay well and had given not only me but Mam, Dad and Sarah love and support when they needed it. I gave my sister Sarah a special present, as a token of how much I really love her, even though we do fight.

The only people not to turn up were the DISCO. I could see Mam and Dad were not very pleased, and they asked someone from the Cricket Club if there was any music we could put on while we waited for the disco to turn up. They did manage to find some music, if you can call it that! It sounded about two hundred years old and was obviously performed by people who still wore flared trousers! Anyway, Dad decided to say a few words. I suppose like most kids there are times when I get really annoyed with my mam and dad, but there are some times when I am really proud of them and I think I must have the best mam and dad in the world – and this was one of those days. Dad thanked everyone for turning up and told them the party wasn't for me, Sarah, Mam or himself, but for everyone who was out there. He thanked the doctors and nurses, the

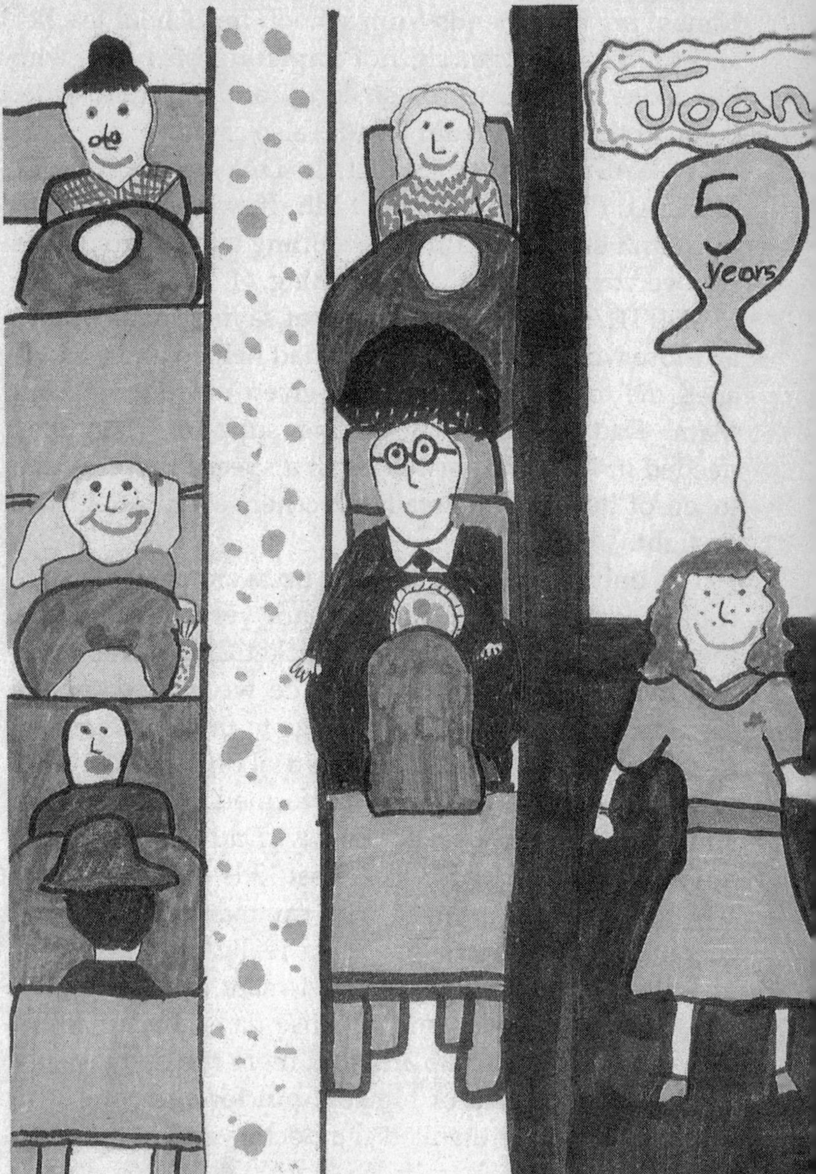
Joan
5
years

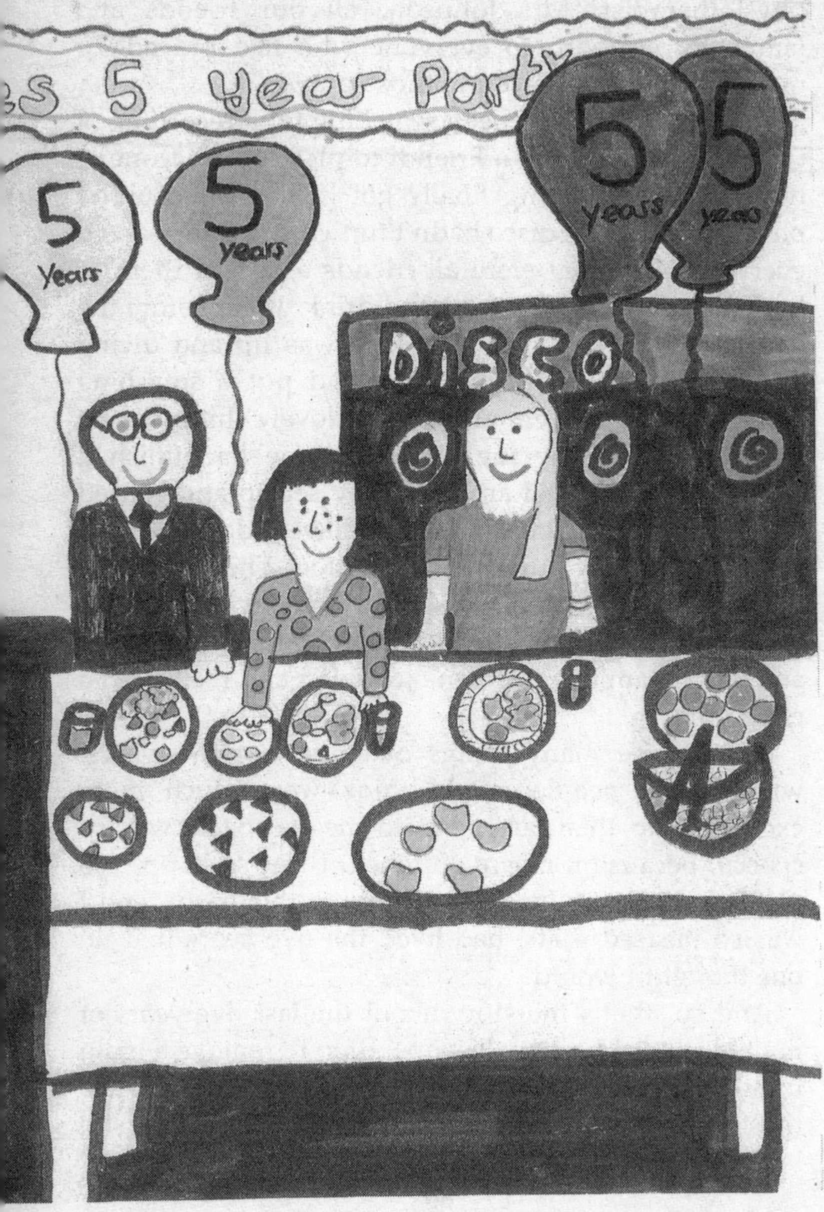
es 5 year Party
5 Years
5 years
5 years
5 years
DISCO

physiotherapist, Mrs Johnson, all our friends and family for support, to everyone who had prayed for me, and God for answering those prayers.

For months we had been searching for a recording of 'Thank You for Being a Friend' to play for everyone at the party and, having finally got hold of it, couldn't play it because the disco hadn't turned up! Dad assured everyone that they were all friends and told them to help themselves to the food and drink. Well, before the words had left his lips, everyone was up and diving towards the food. Jan and Val had put a smashing spread on, there were all kinds of lovely things to eat and fortunately, by the time everyone had finished eating, the disco had arrived. They set up and started to play music we could finally all have a dance to. We were able to play our special song too. The rest of the day was fantastic. Jeff Banks was up dancing with his wife Sue and his children, Tommy was up with Jack and all my family – everyone joined in and really had a good time.

I had done many things over the last five years, which most people would think were much more exciting than this party, but to me the party was so special, because it meant so much. I was so happy, so pleased that everyone could come to this party, and I was so pleased that I had lived the five years that no one thought I would.

And so, that's the story about the last five years of my life, since I had my last operation to remove a brain tumour. It's not going to end there, because now I have the future in front of me. I know the doctors are still not convinced that I am well and some feel the tumour may come back at some stage. So what? I am OK now! And I am looking forward to the future, even though I don't know what it holds.

I'M BETTER

Some people are very clever

I'm better

Some people can run very fast

I'm better

Some people are great at maths

I'm better

Some people are really good at swimming

I'm better

I'm not really showing off because no matter

what people say

Once I was very poorly but now with God's help I

can say

I'M BETTER

I don't know what I would like to be; I would like to be famous, though I doubt I will be. I suppose if Stock, Aitken and Waterman fancy a real challenge I could be a singer but I doubt that too. I would like to be a famous authoress, but I don't know if that will ever happen. I suppose I would just like to make a difference. For someone to say 'Joanne Gillespie did that!' or 'If it hadn't been for Joanne Gillespie, we'd never have been able to do that.' I don't want to sound big-headed, it's just that I think if you don't want something badly enough, then it's not really worth having. Before I go I would just like to say one other thing: if you've been ill like me and there has been something wrong with you, like when I was fat and lost all my hair, and you don't feel like going outside or joining in, scared that people will laugh at you, well *go* outside, and if people laugh, ignore them – why should ignorant people like that spoil your life? You only have one life so enjoy it, live it to the full. If you're reading this and you've never been ill, then please, when you see people in the street and they are walking funny or they have a twisted arm or something unusual about them, please don't laugh, because those people are much tougher than you. Would *you* be able to walk down the street with no hair, or with some other disablement? If friends you are with laugh, don't join in just for the fun of it, try to convince them they are wrong. Put yourself in their situation and try to imagine just how much effort that person is having to make, just to walk down that street or to see people looking and laughing or staring. It's the stares that sometimes hurt more than anything else!

These people are heroes and they deserve your encouragement. Please don't make them look fools!

Well, that's about it. I hope you've enjoyed my book, and that maybe someone has been helped by it. I know that I've done a lot of things that most people will never do, but that's not what's important. What's important is that I've stayed alive five years longer than most people expected. Without that I would have achieved nothing.

So, be positive – you can do it – don't just think, 'Well, I've had the operation, so I should be OK.' The doctors and nurses do their bit, but then it's up to you. Tell yourself, 'I want to be better, I want to walk, or dance or sing or paint or anything.' Don't just hope it happens – MAKE IT HAPPEN! It might not always be easy but remember those are the days when God is trusting in you to be strong.

I hope your life is long and filled with love and laughter and happiness. GOODBYE AND GOD BLESS.

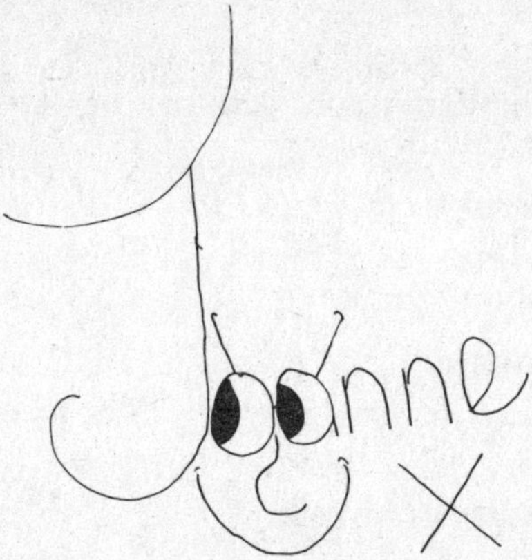

THANKS

Thanks God for listening to me, all those times when I wanted to talk to you,

Even though I go on a bit,

Thanks for helping me when I asked

And thanks for laughter

Thank you God for Michael Jackson, loud music, ballet and snowflakes

For strawberries and Doctors and Snowmen and Scarecrows

and even some dentists!

Thanks for families and friends and all the things I don't understand

Though some may be painful like war and death and hunger

I still thank you because you are giving me the chance to help others

And when its time to put away all the things you gave me

Please God, don't let me say 'Why'

Let me say THANKS

Monica Porter

DREAMS AND DOORWAYS £3.99

Turning Points in the Lives of Famous People

Where did Terry Pratchett's amazing imagination come from? Why did Edwina Currie choose politics? When did fashion first catch the eye of Bruce Oldfield? (Or was it the other way round?) And can you guess which of the names below invented the disco?

Monica Porter talks to twenty-seven people, for whom the doorways of success have now opened wide, about the dreams of their early years.

DOUGLAS ADAMS • BONNIE LANGFORD • VIVIANA DURANTE
SIR ROBIN DAY • HENRY COOPER • JUDY BLUME • ROSHAN SETH
EDINA RONAY • JACK STRAW • PENELOPE LIVELY
BRUCE OLDFIELD • CHRISTOPHER CHATAWAY
DAME BARBARA CARTLAND • NAIM ATTALLAH • QUENTIN BLAKE
PETER SCUDAMORE • KEN LIVINGSTONE • SUSAN HAMPSHIRE
ANDREW SACHS • BISHOP ROY WILLIAMSON
DAVE PROWSE • TERRY PRATCHETT • RABBI JULIA NEUBERGER
FATIMA WHITBREAD • SIR JIMMY SAVILE
TIMMY MALLETT • EDWINA CURRIE